Ike & Marybeth –

Thank you for all your support.

Especially your friendship –

Thank you with all my Heart –

Jim 11-22-72

# The 7 Steps To Personal Power

# THE 7 STEPS TO PERSONAL POWER

## Creating Opportunities Within

James M. Thomas, Jr., Ph.D.

**Health Communications, Inc.**
**Deerfield Beach, Florida**

**Library of Congress Cataloging-in-Publication Data**

Thomas, James M.
    The 7 steps to personal power: creating opportunities within/
James M. Thomas.
        p.     cm.
    ISBN 1-55874-241-7
    1. Self-actualization (Psychology) 2. Self-control. 3. Chakras.
I. Title.   II. Title: Seven steps to personal power.
BF637.S4T49   1992                                        92-20689
158'.1—dc20                                                    CIP

©1992 James M. Thomas, Jr.
ISBN 1-55874-241-7

Publisher: Health Communications, Inc.
            3201 S.W. 15th Street
            Deerfield Beach, Florida 33442-8190

*Cover design by Iris T. Slones*

# Dedication

To my loving wife, Sally, whose support and strength have been my inspiration, not only in what I accomplish, but in who I AM. . . . The greatest opportunity I ever exercised.

# Acknowledgments

I wish to thank my friends and family who affirmed me when I doubted, prodded me when I hesitated and labored with me when the day seemed too long.

I appreciate these special people: Meredith Thomas, Charles Danley, Linda Cowley, Jim and Carolyn Munger, Nancy Terrill, Alma Hopkins, Kevin McAfee and Debbie Sharp for their efforts and awareness.

Additional thanks to Linda Cowley for her time and determination as technical editor.

Barbara Nichols, Chief Editor of Health Communications, and her assistant, Gail Chernoff, and Marie Stilkind, Senior Editor, contributed immeasurably to the final editing and arrangement of content within the book. Barbara helped by acting as both my clarifier and conscience and challenged me to focus my ideas at a deeper level. Thank you, Barbara, for all you have done and especially for the "writing lessons."

# Contents

Prologue ........................................................... xi

Introduction ...................................................... xiii

1. Become Your Own Consultant ........................... 1

2. How We Stop Ourselves .................................... 21

3. Claim The Power Within ................................... 29

4. Create What You Need ...................................... 41

5. Cultivate Emotional Balance ............................. 61

6. Set Your Heart On Your Goal ........................... 83

7. Go With Your Inner Voice ................................ 101

8. Know The Power Within ................................... 127

9. Connect With The Divine ................................. 153

10. Taking The 7 Steps To Personal Power ............. 169

11. Are You Out Of Options? ................................. 177

Appendix ........................................................... 187

Bibliography ...................................................... 189

The seven steps often appear in magical philosophy. In the mid-sixteenth century, alchemist Raymond Lully's book, *On the Ascent*, shows the seven steps to eternal wisdom as stones, fire, plants, animals, man, the starry heavens and the angels. He wrote, "The man of wisdom will attain higher and higher degrees of knowledge until he will be able to apprehend the sublime and the eternal." In the seventeenth century, Heinrich Khunrath's *Amphitheatre of Eternal Wisdom* depicted wise men ascending the seven steps before they reach the hidden light of wisdom.

"All of the ancient systems I have studied have one thing in common," says Dr. James M. Thomas, Jr. "They lead to the Divine. The highest expression of humanness is connection with our Divine source." In this book, Dr. Thomas, a psychologist and Episcopal lay preacher, has turned to the chakra system for practical guidance in finding a path to personal empowerment. "The path is intrinsically there in each of us," Dr. Thomas says. "We're on it whether we choose it or not. We have been given seven great abilities to help us live consciously and meaningfully. We can ignore them or we can develop them."

In working with private patients and corporate clients who want to make changes, Dr. Thomas reports a high rate of success when people become aware of their intrinsic powers and learn how to use them.

We hope this interesting system will help you understand your great inner gifts and use them in an inspired way.

                                              The Editors

# Introduction

For more than 20 years in my practice of psychotherapy I have worked with clients who come to my office for help when they feel overwhelmed, unable to deal with the problems of life effectively. They display symptoms of stress and may feel inadequate and underpowered. Some feel they have painted themselves into a corner, stuck in dull marriages or go-nowhere jobs. They would like to improve things but feel discouraged and dispirited. Nothing seems to work and they want help in straightening out their lives.

I know these feelings well.

I felt completely overwhelmed when I was a young captain in the Vietnam War and was diagnosed with Hodgkin's disease — cancer of the lymph nodes. We knew less about cancer at that time than we do now, and I thought I had been given a death sentence. I was sent back to a veteran's hospital in the States where the diagnosis was confirmed and arrangements for a medical discharge were made. Before my discharge came through, I left the hospital feeling pretty well. I hopped a plane bound for Korea — it was the time of the Pueblo crisis and we were shorthanded there. Perhaps I could help out. Staying busy would at least keep my mind off my situation.

What happened to me on Easter Sunday morning on the outskirts of Seoul can only be described as an unbidden miracle of spiritual healing. Spontaneously I fell into a trance as an enormous surge of power raced through me, igniting the energy of my body. The Spirit of God, the Holy Spirit, the Great Spirit, the Universal Energy, the Self of All, call it what you will, mobilized every fiber of my being and I knew I was cured. At the same time a voice, sounding very much like my own, told me to become a psychologist and help people. This was a career I had never considered.

When I got back to the States, I no longer had Hodgkin's disease. The diagnosis was downgraded to sarcoidosis, a much lesser disease of the lymph system. I had no symptoms then nor have I ever experienced any recurrence of Hodgkin's disease or sarcoidosis in the 25 years since.

Experiencing the miracle of such radical positive change gave me confidence that I could help others have their own miracles. I went ahead and studied psychology. I have also made a lifelong study of comparative religion to understand God as well as I could and to search for understanding of ways people throughout history have sought access to their Creator. I find that many people who experience miracles in their lives become seekers of spiritual truth, interested in learning about different spiritual systems.

I am a Christian and a lay preacher in the Episcopal church yet have great respect for other belief systems. The paths to God are many and diverse, and knowledge of them creates a spiritual richness that enhances our experience of connection to others, to our Creator and to the power within bestowed on us by an all-powerful God of love.

The theory of the seven steps to personal power evolved through the exciting adventure of helping others unravel mysteries of their own minds. It brings my knowledge of science and theology together with my understanding of the ancient theory of chakras, or subtle energy centers, believed to exist in every person. In Oriental cultures, from Hindu to Buddhist, these centers have been known for thousands of years and form the basis for many healing systems in use now, from acupuncture to Ayurvedic medicine. The seven chakras represent seven subtle powers of mind. Taken together, they suggest a dynamic unity of body, mind and spirit.

It was many years after that rosy Easter near Seoul when I learned of the chakras, but I recognized immediately their similarity to the miracle of healing I received that day. The movement of the chakra energies was an experience of energy circulating through my body and healing me on that fateful morning.

I believe anyone seeking to expand their awareness of their personal power can benefit by learning about this ancient system. It is not my intention to present a comprehensive look at such subtle wisdom here, but to build on the primary idea that human beings have seven intrinsic powers of mind that we can develop to our advantage. In this book I combine information from the chakra system with modern psychological principles. The result is a useful workable system I call the seven steps to personal power.

When we talk about personal power, it is important to understand that we are not discussing power over anyone or anything other than ourselves. Personal power is the ability to generate opportunities from the creative resources within us which are consistent with our goals and values.

My intention is to bring you deeper understanding of the powers within and a way to work with them. Though much information in this book is thousands of years old, it is translated here as an intrinsic part of a modern model for self-directed change.

I suggest ways to access the most powerful, caring and creative consultant ever — your own inner wisdom and problem-solving skills. The only requirement for employing this great assistant is for you to approach your thoughts, feelings and discoveries with self-respect. Be courageous! Be open to your own suggestions and resources.

I hope you find this way of inner learning useful in your day-to-day life.

*James M. Thomas, Jr., Ph.D.*
*Ponca City, Oklahoma*

# 1 Become Your Own Consultant

Many times in your life you may have wished for a personal advisor, therapist or manager — someone who really understood your needs, who cared for you and gave good advice on what to do next and how to do it. You may have a crisis or a point of choice where you feel stuck and want more good options. Maybe you feel there are too many decisions, too little time and energy and you need help fast. You might be bothered by a recurring symptom or unhealthy behavior pattern. You might even feel that you are stuck in a place you have been stuck many times before.

Which job?

Which person? What about my parents? My kids? My spouse?

Where will the money, energy, support, leadership come from?

What is my next move and how do I get the help I need?
What is my best option?
Where are the real opportunities?

It might seem as if you need a collection of experts to answer these questions. The truth is, the best advice you can get is within your own consciousness. Your inner consultant is wise and caring, has your best interests at heart and already knows the best choices you can make. Though it lies dormant in most of us, we can, in effect, hire this informed, caring advisor. We can learn to access our personal power, our inner source of creativity, and put it to work for us. Years of work with my patients and corporate clients confirms my belief in the efficacy of our inner consultant.

## How It Began
* * * * * * *

Very early in our lives we trusted ourselves enough to really pay attention to our inner creative resources. Our own thoughts and feelings were of paramount importance to us. We instinctively knew we should follow the subtle urgings of intuition. But in the process of growing up we came to distrust and disregard the inner voice that serves to guide our actions and impulses. When we innocently and earnestly wanted to please a parent, teacher or other significant person in our young lives, we internalized the criticism we received. As a result, we became skeptical of our creative impulses and inner guidance.

We learned to ignore the subtle signals of our inherent wisdom, to censor the wellspring of opportunities that arose in our minds and hearts. Now we are left with the legacy of shutting down our inner guidance systems. We feel the effect of this shutdown when faced with critical decisions. We wait and hope for inspiration or a surge of divinity to activate our energy systems and bring us back to balance.

In a very real sense, our opinions of our abilities are molded by memory. Did we succeed or fail in the past? We become trapped in nostalgia, our attention focused on how it used to be, on what we did then. We become confused in mind and in action.

## Creating Our Own Opportunities
* * * * * * *

Almost everyone who comes to my office says, in one way or another, that they want more choices and the increased ability to carry them out. When I suggest to them that they are the creators of their own opportunities, they hesitate. The idea seems familiar, but they are not sure they believe it. They are not sure they believe in themselves.

No matter what your past experience has been, I know you can affect the opportunities that present themselves to you now. You can actually create an array of possible outcomes when you learn to use your personal power.

Personal power does not mean having power or control over others. It means possessing the resources to shape your own destiny by seizing the opportunities that exist in the present.

The best opportunities are those that arise from the depths of our minds and hearts. They are the product of appropriate beliefs coupled with sincere respect for the good intentions of our unconscious minds. Our power to master ourselves and our behavior does not stem so much from developing self-control as from accessing many levels of inner awareness and allowing communication and co-operation between them.

Sufis say consciousness is like a lake. The mind is the surface of the heart, and the heart is the depth of the mind. If we skip a stone over the surface of the water, we learn superficial knowledge about the pond; if we wish to learn what is at the bottom of the pond, we must throw the stone directly into its depths. In the same way, the depth of the answer we receive from ourselves is in direct proportion to the depth of the question we ask.

This book is about the process of self-inquiry and self-empowerment. It presents step-by-step methods for gaining information from deep within our own creative resources and putting it to work in our lives.

## Identifying Where We're Stuck
* * * * * * *

There are many different levels to our psychological selves and they are constantly interacting, working as parts of our energy system. It is as if we have a family of characters inside who have the common problems and frailties of most families. They may be in harmony or in conflict, but they are always influencing one another.

A deep and difficult truth to accept is that *every part of us has the intention of protecting us and getting us out of situations in which we may falter.* Over the years I have observed these good and positive intentions in literally every person I've worked with. Even if behavior is bad, malevolent or harmful to self, the intention of the part of the personality activating behavior is to protect the individual. The protection may manifest as getting us out of a scrape or retreating from some potentially overwhelming responsibility.

One client complained that he never had enough money. Every financial success was followed by a failure. As we worked together to reach the depths of his problem, we uncovered an internal belief that money would hurt him. He was a creative person whose natural thought process was very visual. He had little trouble accessing a literal inner family of tight-lipped, hard-working pioneers. They were afraid money would turn him into a hard-drinking, fast-living cowboy. How could he get around their stern inner judgment which had been manifesting in his life as a kind of fear of success? I convinced him that the inner pioneers really were on his side, cared about him and had his best interests at heart. As they understood it, they were protecting him. He needed to thank them, to work with them, to help them understand that his intentions were good, too, and that his success would benefit all of them.

Not all of us come to understand our inner selves as visually as this creative person did, but all of us can learn to understand and trust our inner wisdom. The important thing to accept is the deep and difficult truth — that every part of us has the intention of protecting us and getting us out of situations in which we may falter.

I began to understand the inner powers of the mind in the 1960s when I was diagnosed with Hodgkin's disease — cancer of the lymph nodes. As far as I knew, it was a death sentence, but instead of giving in to fate, I unconsciously mobilized every resource I had to cure the incurable.

I was a young officer stationed at Fairchild Air Force Base near Spokane where I was involved with liaison between the 15th Air Force and AT&T, a major government contractor. It was an interesting job and I planned to continue working for AT&T when I left the service.

I was sent to Vietnam where I was communications officer for a squadron of KC-135s, air-to-air refuelers. We had been flying through clouds of Agent Orange, and when I became ill with a lung and lymph condition, I thought that might be the cause.

The Air Force sent me back to their hospital near St. Louis, and I was diagnosed with Hodgkin's disease. It was cancer, the dreaded C word, and I was too young to have it. I had a wife, a promising future in civilian life with AT&T — and my time was running out. After recuperating for several weeks I began to feel well enough to be discharged from the hospital and recuperate at home while waiting for my medical discharge. Rather than sitting around worrying, I decided to jump on a plane bound for Korea. The Pueblo incident had just occurred and the U.S.

needed everyone they could get in Korea without taking
them from active duty in 'Nam. I had nothing to lose.

In Seoul a tough top sergeant befriended me and asked
me to accompany him and his friends to an orphanage
run by the Methodist Church on the outskirts of town. It
was Easter and the children needed a treat. I needed a
treat, too, and a trip to the orphanage had special appeal.
I had grown up in the Methodist Church and as a boy had
ambitions to become a missionary. At least I could fulfill
that part of my life plan for a day.

Some of us decided to hide eggs for an Easter surprise
for the children. At daybreak on Easter Sunday I was in
an open field, hiding eggs under bushes. As the rosy light
of dawn grew bright I suddenly experienced an incredible
shift of consciousness and went into what I can only describe as a trance. In this different reality, a new kind of
energy circulated through my body and I knew I had been
touched by the unseen hand of God. This vivid burst of
energy was followed by a voice, which seemed to be my
own, telling me to become a psychotherapist and devote
my life to helping people.

I was bursting with intense feelings of love and gratitude.

I felt that God had talked to me and I knew everything
would be all right. I believed that I had received a healing.
I'd seen some miraculous healings before — my mother
and her father and brothers had all been gifted spiritual
healers back in Missouri — but never had anything like
this happened to me. When I got back to the United
States, I went back to the hospital. No trace of cancer
could be found and all symptoms were alleviated. The
doctors changed my diagnosis to sarcoidosis, a lesser disease of the lymph system, though I had no symptoms of
anything — just some residual scarring of my lungs and
lymph system.

The incident in Seoul was a miracle and it changed my
life forever. I had my mission and knew just what to do.
Becoming a psychotherapist had never entered my mind

but I honored that very clear directive I received. I don't know what would have happened if I hadn't, but I do know I have not had a recurrence of Hodgkin's disease nor sarcoidosis and have been symptom-free for almost 25 years.

When the mysterious power that cured my cancer suggested I become a psychotherapist and help people, I kept the bargain. Years later when I saw the film *Field of Dreams* with Kevin Costner, I was struck by the similarities between that story and my own. Costner was told by an improbable voice, "If you build it, they will come," and the story revolves around his struggle to acknowledge and act on the message. In the end he builds that baseball field in the middle of a cornfield against all odds, and people flock to it. When you begin to do inner work, it's crucial to keep the promises you make to yourself.

## The Seven Steps To Personal Power: A System That Works
* * * * * * *

My seven-step system of self-empowerment has been honed during 20 years of work as a psychologist, and I know it works. It is a productive formula for living in which you apply basic time-tested principles of health and wellness to your daily life. You can use this system to improve the way you deal with all of life's challenges, both great and small. It works to climb literal or metaphoric mountains or to glide over life's little speed bumps. The seven steps can help you pass a test, give a speech, achieve inner composure, select a mate or choose a new and different life path.

My theory brings the chakra system, taught by Eastern cultures for thousands of years, into alignment with Western psychology. By combining these two powerful thought streams, we enhance our ability to find peace, harmony and a happier life. The seven steps in my system correlate with the seven chakras of the ancients, which represent seven distinct powers of mind. You can use the energy of these seven powers to get the best from yourself and your relationships and to find solutions within your deep, inner center of wisdom.

## Ancient And Not-So-Ancient Ideas On Human Development
* * * * * * *

For the most part, Westerners are educated to apply the power of logic and reason to every problem. Scholars in several ancient civilizations cultivated more intuitive or experiential knowledge. In the healing arts, some Oriental cultures still rely on theories of energy systems developed thousands of years ago. The origin of these theories has been lost for centuries in the desert sands or steaming jungles, but it is likely that the idea evolved from a prehistoric healer's sensitivity to subtle body energy.

The subtle energies of the body and mind may have been discovered spontaneously in several locations. Flint needles dating from 7000 to 5000 B.C. have been found, indicating that Neolithic humans practiced pain control similar to modern day acupuncture which utilizes pathways of subtle energy.

Professor Rhys Davids describes Buddha's doctrine of *Dhammachakkappavattana Sutta* which involved energy centers called chakras, named after royal chariot wheels, or "chakkas" in Sanskrit. Traditional yoga philosophy refers to chakras and describes them as subtle force centers which vitalize and control human development. And the *Nei Ching*, a 24-volume set of wisdom attributed to Huang Ti, the "Yellow Emperor" who ruled China from 2697 to 2597 B.C., refers to the existence of *chi*, the vital body energy.

The writings of Hermes Trismegistus of ancient Egypt, a contemporary of Abraham of the Old Testament, included the Kybalion, a set of seven basic doctrines. It set forth the "transmutation" of vibrations of the body into mental energy which helped one to transcend from a humble student to a master of understanding. The Vedas, holy writings from fifth and sixth century India, discuss evolution of human consciousness from infancy to old age in terms of theoretical "platforms," which correspond to different levels of body development. The highest platform is one of spiritual bliss.

In most old paintings of Christian saints and other religious art throughout the world, a halo or ring of light surrounding the head of the holy person is depicted, denoting holiness or some kind of spiritual ascension.

The idea of body energy or light representing the ultimate in spiritual development or holiness is an almost universal symbol. From primitive man to the ancient Egyptians, Hebrews, Chinese, Indians and Europeans, the idea of energy centers within the human body is associated with healing and growth. Today medical advances that hold promise for the future include biofeedback, psychoimmunology and bioenergy techniques. The idea of using the energy systems of the human body for healing and growth is as relevant now as it has been for thousands of years.

At the core of my seven steps, you will find the idea that we operate at different levels of consciousness which correspond to the chakras. The dynamic interaction of these levels determines the state, or stage, of our development.

Those who are familiar with the seven chakras hold that we develop physically, emotionally, mentally and spiritually as energy moves upwards through the system. The chakras are located in a vertical line up and down our bodies as in the drawing on the next page.

The first, or base, chakra is located at the very bottom of the spine. The other chakras, numbered two through seven, are located progressively upwards to the last, or seventh, chakra which is located at the crown of the head.

Chakras distribute energy appropriately throughout the body to facilitate growth and body harmony. They supply energy to any part of the body when it is needed, especially when disease is present. This system controls every body organ as well as whole systems of body functioning. Every chakra is associated with different organs and characteristics.

Organs/Glands/Senses
Colors/Odors
Types of Energy/Body Systems
Stages of Development
Personalities

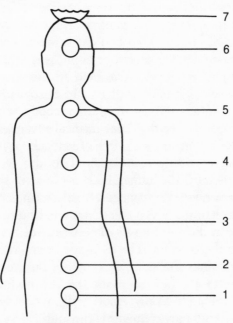

**Figure 1.1. The Chakras**

In this system of thinking, almost everything about us originates from the inner workings of these chakras. If we learn to live in a balanced way, energy ascends and as time goes by, we become more wise, loving and more spiritual. Each chakra has a spiritual splendor, waiting to reveal itself to us.

The more open we remain to life and the changes life brings, the more energy will flow unimpeded, bringing health to every aspect of our being. Illness can be viewed as a blockage of energy pathways or an uneven distribution of energy throughout the body. When the body is out of balance, our perceptions, thoughts and feelings are diminished. We are more vulnerable to stress, malfunction of every body system, and eventually, disease.

Because the chakras are total energy systems, they are connected with our psychological states as well as our physical health. Too much energy causes confusion, too little causes atrophy. Either way, growth is delayed or stunted as it is in early childhood trauma, such as sexual abuse. If overstimulation occurs in the sexual area, energy tends to accumulate in the sacral chakra and the child becomes "sexualized." Overstimulation may cause problems with sexual behavior, feelings and self-image.

I had a client whose father was a gynecologist. As a teen he begged his father to allow him to observe surgery. The effects on him were the same as in a situation of direct sexual abuse. The young man was overstimulated in a negative way. Witnessing women's bodies being cut open in the sexual area caused him to be impotent for much of his life. He received too much stimulation before he was ready to integrate the experience. (He was also stimulated in a positive way by developing an understanding of surgery.)

A similar scenario takes place when traumatic experiences of all kinds overwhelm victims' ability to cope. The chakra model helps us to understand and treat post-traumatic stress syndrome in trauma victims. Essentially we take stress off these victims, make sure they rest and become strong enough to allow the energy level to reshift and reach homeostasis again. (Taking yourself out of a tough situation is the opposite of brainwashing.) Then we regress the clients, get them to go back into the experience again. They don't really want to get out of it because of the pain and uncertainty. Not pushing them too hard or too fast is very important.

These techniques were first thought out while working with Vietnam vets. It is a very delicate process to remain open to experience while containing our stress within controllable limits so we can avoid being overwhelmed. Becoming sensitive to the subtle energies of the chakras enables us to find the balance point and never push ourselves or our clients too far.

The chakras run up the midline of the body. Each one regulates a certain psychophysical system. Rather than saying simply that the second, or sacral chakra, influences just sexual glands, we need to understand that each chakra is in correspondence with an entire system. In the case of the second chakra, the system involves the ovaries or testes (the physical organs and glands of sexuality), the lower back, the reproductive forces and the sexual energy. The sexual energy is also, in its more refined aspects, the energy of creativity of all kinds, whether it is directed toward creating a new life, a sonnet, a dance, a computer program or a company. In the case of the second chakra, even if the organs are removed, the system remains intact at a more subtle level.

The following chart of the major chakras shows their names and locations, the psychophysical system they correspond to and the type of energy and color associated with each chakra. You need to grasp this ancient model in order to understand how its truths apply to our contemporary model of character development.

## How The Seven Chakras And Seven Steps Work Together
★ ★ ★ ★ ★ ★ ★

Consider the seven steps as a path toward enhancement of your personal power, of your ability to attain your dreams. The steps correlate with the seven chakras and provide a bridge between wisdom of the ancients and the "how to" of modern psychology. They help you transcend the problems and limits of the present and generate those all-important creative opportunities for the future. Taking these steps may even lead us to understand that we are personally called to play a more important role in life than we have ever dreamed of, well above and beyond our present situation.

### Table 1.1.

| Chakra Name | Location | System | Energy | Color | Organ/Gland |
|---|---|---|---|---|---|
| 7. Crown | Crown | Spirit | Spirit | White | Higher Brain |
| 6. Head | Forehead | Brain | Thought | Indigo | Eye/Ear/Senses |
| 5. Throat | Neck | Speech | Communication | Blue | Lung/Thyroid |
| 4. Heart | Chest | Blood | Life | Green | Heart/Thymus |
| 3. Solar | Stomach | Digest | Emotion | Yellow | Digestive |
| 2. Sacral | Lower Back | Reproduction | Creative | Orange | Gonads |
| 1. Base | Base of Spine | Force | Will | Red | Spinal |

The seven steps involve . . .

- A thorough understanding of ourselves
- An awareness of the predictable changes that are likely to occur in our lives
- An ability to predict reasonably the probable outcome of future events which come about in the natural process of maturing and growing to trust ourselves.

---

## Table 1.2.

## How The Old And New Models Correspond

| Chakra | Personal Power Step |
|---|---|
| 7. Crown <br> The top of the head, energy of the spirit, connection to the Divine | Connect With The Divine |
| 6. Forehead <br> The brain, focused thoughts and ideas | Know The Power Within |
| 5. Throat <br> Speech, expression, communication | Go With Your Inner Voice |
| 4. Heart <br> Heart-centered Emotions of Love and Forgiveness | Set Your Heart On Change |
| 3. Solar Plexus <br> Emotional energy, taking in and assimilating energy from the environment | Cultivate Emotional Balance |
| 2. Sacral (Lower Back) <br> Sexual, generative, creative energy | Create What You Need |
| 1. Base (Coccyx or Lower Spine) <br> Force, will, power to take a stand, make decisions | Claim The Power Within |

---

The energy of life ascends in a natural flow as we grow. It is not like an elevator going up, leaving one floor before it gets to the next. Rather, it is a subtle current that connects our powers, sometimes emphasizing one, sometimes another, and eventually synthesizing them into an integrated, effective whole. If we are damaged in a particular area, like the boy who helped his gynecologist father, the flow of energy through that area may be uneven. We need to become aware of our deficiencies and get the energy flowing again.

In brief, here is how the seven steps work. In subsequent chapters we go into each step at length, but it helps to have an overview at the beginning.

## The First Step To Personal Power: Claim The Power Within

We begin to claim our power when we understand the significance of our beliefs. Your belief system is exactly and precisely what guides and directs your life, both consciously and unconsciously. It is the foundation of experience, just as a basement is the foundation of a house. We create our own reality, then unconsciously attempt to live out our belief of what is going to happen. This process works in subtle ways.

When we decide to take over direction of our lives, we enlist the power of our will, which is the power of the first chakra. Directing our lives involves focusing the direction of our inner thoughts and actions. To follow through we need to access our creative, unconscious resources, find ways to affirm our abilities and reinforce and nurture positive opportunities.

Unless we fully understand the potent concept of engaging and believing in our own will, setting a new direction remains difficult if not impossible. Appreciating the significance of our beliefs is the first step we take to bring positive possibilities into our lives. An act of will is the basis for change of beliefs, and the energy of will moves upward through the entire system. Getting your will to work for you may be easier than you think.

## The Second Step To Personal Power: Create What You Need

The second step uses our power to create. It involves understanding how our unconscious mind generates opportunities and possibilities for positive change. What could be more creative than giving birth to a new way of life for ourselves? This step emphasizes the concept of positive orientation. If we create negative ideas, such as, "This probably won't work," we're almost guaranteed a negative result. Whatever it is, it has little chance for success if it is sent out under a negative banner. The words we choose when we speak with ourselves and others naturally help or hinder our ability to create positive opportunities. Like the baby elephant who steps on her own nose, some of us unwittingly get in our own way. We need to learn to stop sabotaging ourselves. And on the positive side of the ledger, we can learn to free our inner abilities to chart and hold a positive course. Generating creativity is an ongoing dynamic process.

## The Third Step To Personal Power: Cultivate Emotional Balance

Our real energy to change comes from the power of the third chakra, our emotions. Emotions determine congruency or lack of congruency between our inner beliefs and outer actions. Negative emotions, which you may not even be aware of, can keep you from believing you can do your best and prevent you from acting in your own best interests.

Your potential for taking charge of your future is directly proportional to the level of congruency, or similarity, that exists between your inner beliefs and outer actions. When we are congruent and live out our innermost beliefs in our day-to-day lives, we tend to be receptive and open to positive opportunities. Congruency leads us to the experience of "following our bliss," and to being able to actualize our potential for well-being and service to others. It is specifically the cooperative interaction between conscious and unconscious levels of mind that directs us to become focused and committed to our goals. Lack of cooperation between these levels of mind signifies a lack of personal integration. If we are not operating from high levels of integrity, how can we follow through on our goals and purposes?

## The Fourth Step To Personal Power: Set Your Heart On Change

The energy of the fourth chakra is naturally directed to love and forgiveness. Perception and understanding are heightened in anyone who becomes able to forgive and live without resentment, anger or bitterness. Forgiveness allows us to keep moving and growing in positive directions.

If we lack the ability to forgive, we may find ourselves blind to our best intentions. To set our minds and hearts on our creative goals we need to clear out the negative emotions we hold toward those who inflicted harm on us. Without forgiveness, which leads to a loving and accepting attitude, we place great limitations on ourselves and block our efforts to achieve positive results. Many people are blocked at the level of their hearts, caught in perpetual states of undischarged grief. There they remain stuck and immobilized, blaming others for their condition. When we use the energy of the heart chakra, we can move through necessary steps of forgiving ourselves and others.

## The Fifth Step To Personal Power: Go With Your Inner Voice

The fifth step incorporates many small steps inward to determine meaning and essence in our lives and relationships. The process includes communicating with a deep inner source and living life in a kind of partnership with that source. We spontaneously receive and respond to information gleaned from our creative resources.

This step might be considered a speed-shift into the activity of change. The fifth chakra, located at the level of the throat, is the natural energy of communication. It represents the force we need to fully commit to a new course of action. When we can proudly tell ourselves and others of our new intentions, our probability of following through increases. When I decided to write this book, for example, it was necessary for me to bring my intention to the level of expression. Until I could say clearly to myself and others what I was intending, the task could not be accomplished.

Being able to express our power through communication is especially significant at times when change is natural and inevitable. When we grow into new phases of life, such as our middle years, the power of the fifth chakra helps us to refine our expression and claim new interests. Often our inner being chooses more refined cultural and spiritual interests at that time. If the ascending energy of the lower chakras is not blocked, it naturally breaks through to the level of the fifth chakra communicating to us our need to change and grow.

If we are not aware that such a process will happen, we may adamantly hold on to our old lives and may even die trying to live out a purpose which we have outgrown. On the positive side, many of us experience it as a calling to a new place or lifestyle. Others may view it negatively, much as they view aging of the physical body. We can accept predictable changes and discover new meaning, or we can retreat into boredom or chaos.

There are two situations which may thrust us into this stage of transformation before we are ready. First, achieving our earlier goals can be surprisingly traumatic. Where do you go after you've arrived? A friend told me he had a rush of almost suicidal depression the day he realized he had achieved his goal of becoming a millionaire. The other major disruption which hurls us into change occurs after an intensely personal crisis, such as loss of a spouse.

During crises we may attempt to recapture our former lives. The attempt never really works to complete satisfaction. It is important to understand the predictable stages in our life process and equally important to be able to generate new goals and future courses of action.

## The Sixth Step To Personal Power: Know The Power Within

Waking up and really knowing the power within is a process which involves our minds. We must think about what is happening. Bringing the power of thought into sharp focus serves to identify authentic interests while weeding out meaningless internal dialog. At the stage when the sixth chakra is fully open, we feel connected to others, to the land and to some intrinsic purpose. There are definite characteristics that develop when we mature to the point of feeling connected with everything. We merge into a feeling of universality.

When we see events of our lives fitting into an overall plan and know we are doing our best, we attain a state known to philosophers of old as "perfection." We know we are truly alive. We are in focus. We are able to relate intimately to others of all ages and walks of life, leaving behind prejudices and preconceived ideas about their limits.

## The Seventh Step To Personal Power: Connect To The Divine

As we move toward self-mastery we are likely to experience communication with the spiritual source of all life. When we align our strongest inner resources with the highest source, we generate the most creative opportunities for our lives. Attaining this ability to connect at will with the Divine coincides with the opening of the seventh, or crown, chakra, and completes our life's journey toward meaning and purpose. Staying connected with the Divine spirit signifies a high level of self-mastery. When we are open to Divine guidance, our negative qualities seem to burn away and we live an ongoing cleansing process.

As fine sand is to gravel, so spiritual energy is to physical energy. When we live in a state of awakened spirituality, we acquire a fineness of perception and action. We are sensitive, we do the right thing intuitively. We listen and respond to our inner voices. People report learning to expect a daily miracle. And with this delicacy of feeling and perception comes knowing. We attain great inner strength.

Those who successfully find the path to self-empowerment tend to make life look easy. They are relaxed and effective.

## Empowerment Begins
* * * * * * *

I hope this information on the chakra system enlarges your understanding of the interaction of the body and mind.

The chakras and the energy surrounding them are a subject that fills libraries. It is not my intention here to attempt to fully explain the wisdom of the East, but rather, to bring into awareness certain inherent powers of mind that Western culture does not teach us in a unified way.

I've led workshops on this concept for many groups of people, including attorneys (who are extremely analytical), businesspersons, psychologists and Baptist seminarians. By the end of the day, skepticism invariably turns to enthusiasm.

It takes real courage and creativity to see things in a new way and let yourself take in unfamiliar data. But a new world opens up when we increase our tolerance for ambiguity. That which was hidden becomes obvious as we become more perceptive. A century ago the potentials of radium, nuclear energy and outer space were virtually unknown. They were real all along but were unseen and consequently unbelievable to all but a few "dreamers."

Hopefully, taking the seven steps will expand your ability to dream — and make your dreams come true.

CHAPTER

# 2 How We Stop Ourselves

I f we're to empower ourselves to rise above
our limits, we need to get an accurate fix on
what those limits are, and what they appear
to be. Humankind has been unable to get in
touch with all of the abundance and goodness
available in the here and now. We tend to believe in limitation. Physical, mental, emotional
and spiritual obstacles trap us in the status
quo. We're convinced we are less than we are.
Our fears restrain our creativity, our inner
resources and our belief in ourselves.

We can identify five major categories of fear
which bind us to the past. As our journey of
self-empowerment gets underway, we need to
address each of them.

# Fear Of Limitation
* * * * * * *

Limits may be quite real. An American athlete won't win a French National medal in her sport unless she moves to France and becomes a citizen. She is limited by the rules. But if she did comply with the regulations, she might very well win. We can look at factors which limit us and logically decide a course of action.

Fear is harder to deal with. Fear of limitation is only an idea but it stops us. Nothing in the environment can stop us as effectively. I believe that every person knows, yet fails to recognize, his or her innermost desires. The reason we fail to respond to our deep yearnings is our perpetual fear of limitation. We're afraid we won't do it well, win or make it work.

Fear of limitation serves as a powerful injunction against achieving our dreams. It is like a curse cast upon us to keep us from reaching our highest potential. But knowledge of our fear helps us determine means and strategies to get over it.

There are many different types of limits. For example, trauma can continue to thwart us by psychologically, emotionally and spiritually hampering our belief in ourselves and our decision-making process. If we are traumatized physically or emotionally, we come to question our efficacy. We may lose faith in ourselves. Our beliefs can act as a wall or as a gateway to effective coping strategies. Often it is a question of whether we have the mental ability to look beyond present failures. They may be guiding us to future success.

Consider, for example, the lives of successful people. How did they overcome their limitations? They either did not believe in their limitations or knew they could conquer any barrier they encountered. Thomas Edison found nearly 800 ways *not* to make a light bulb before he hit upon the idea which resulted in the predecessor of our modern light bulb. Abraham Lincoln lost nine political races before he won his first election. Lucille Ball was rejected time after time for acting parts before she became the beloved star of *I Love Lucy*. Each of these people had to struggle with the deep, dark face of insecurity and failure *before* they were able to visualize success. It was their mental ability to see beyond their failures that guided them to the success we know them by today.

I have seen many individuals who were at crucial decision points in their lives. These courageous adults often expressed the feeling that they were living between two worlds. They were attempting to bridge past failures with future successes. Yet they felt as if they were barely coping from day to day. Those who eventually become capable of moving their minds to achieve success were those who could reach deep within themselves and cope with their greatest limitation: fear. This limitation has been defined as only a combination of the following elements: **F**(alse) **E**(vidence) **A**(ppearing) **R**(eal). Explaining fear in these terms lets us see it for what it is.

Many people who come to our country for the first time are amazed at how Americans tend to capitalize on fear. It seems to be part of the national character. While I doubt Americans have cornered the market on this limitation, it is interesting to note how advertisers of everything from deodorants to tires to educational programs introduce the notion of fear, or individual insecurity, into their sales campaigns.

After they stimulate our fear of limitation, they offer a foolproof solution with the purchase of their products. President Roosevelt's comment, "The only thing we have to fear is fear itself," suggests a more reasonable cure for our common malady. Still, we may become afraid of being afraid, or *learn* to fear the idea of fear itself.

# The Fear Of Scarcity
* * * * * * *

The basis of fear is actually belief in scarcity. Most psychological and philosophical theories from ancient civilizations to modern times, deal with the concept of fear, directly or indirectly. Every school of human motivation has tactics and techniques for dealing with fear and overcoming its negative effects.

Many people are driven by the belief that if they fail to do something, they will inevitably be needy. Fear of scarcity drives them and holds them back simultaneously. To evalute this fear in my clients, I often ask them to complete this sentence: "If the worst thing that *could* happen to me actually did happen, I would _____" (fill in the blank). Sometimes men and women are astonished by their own responses. Some even comment that the worst possible thing they can think of has already happened. Most people will acknowledge that somehow they would cope with and live through even the most disastrous circumstances in their lives. At the same time they acknowledge what they really want to do is avoid going through the feared circumstances in the first place. Even those who say that the worst thing has already happened to them are still capable of imagining an even worse situation. Then they find themselves in an even more acute emotional state than before.

# Feel Worse Fast
* * * * * * *

During a research study on the nature of fear, I used a stop watch to time how long it actually took people to make themselves feel miserable. The average length of time was 4.3 seconds. I was amazed. I also found that the more creative and bright a person was, the more adept he or she was at self-torture. However, even people with an

I.Q. of about room temperature could still get themselves into a mental funk in less than five seconds very easily!

The most common method to generate self-induced fear is to imagine something they dread happening to them. The rest is accomplished by simply remembering something that happened in the past which made them fearful. In interviewing people about their future or past fears, the fear of scarcity is always evident. Most of us have an idea of what it would take in the future to make us comfortable. This idea is somehow compared to our present situation. Then we generally want more of some things and less of others. Besides thinking about scarcity, we conceptualize an ideal situation, defined as having what we need to deal effectively with life's demands.

The fear of scarcity is taught to us from a very early age. Many of us can recall the motivating power of fear of failing in school or fear of being reprimanded for not pleasing others. One of the major challenges in educational psychology is to determine ways to motivate students with the wish to succeed, rather than the fear of failure. As adults we fear lack of resources, such as money, time, relationships and emotional support. We all occasionally motivate ourselves by the fear of being unable to get something we badly need unless we take some kind of precaution in the present. The "fear of" dynamic and belief in scarcity pervades nearly every aspect of our lives.

## The Fear Of Loss
* * * * * * *

Hoarding material goods and positive emotions is an attempt to cover up our own feelings of vulnerability to catastrophic and sudden loss or depletion of assets. An old truism in salesmanship school tells us the best salesmen "create a need first and then sell the product that fills it." This process is an example of capitalizing on the fear of scarcity.

The new way of selling is to align ourselves with our clients and become partners with them in enhancing their lifestyles through the use of certain products and services.

In acute cases of fear of loss, one's importance is viewed in terms of his or her wealth and status. In this value system, a person with potentially less scarcity is more valuable than one with a potential for future scarcity.

A few years ago a DuPont executive stated his concern about a current attitude about security young people shared. They believed finding security meant taking something away from someone else. He wanted to motivate young people to adopt the idea of creating new options to generate business with better goods and services, rather than thinking of success as taking wealth from one place and putting it in another. Only a generation of young people who could see beyond their own needs could be courageous enough to fulfill the needs of others, he believed. If they only focused on fulfilling imagined scarcity in their own lives, they would not be able to fulfill roles as community leaders.

## The Fear Of Affirmation And Success
\* \* \* \* \* \* \*

Some people lose their ability to affirm others. If we affirm another person, we believe we are taking something away from ourselves. This fear is predicated on the deep belief that intangibles, such as appreciation and love, are limited and exhaustible resources. Sometimes we even get very selfish in showing appreciation and love for ourselves. We fear success for several reasons. People often jokingly say that if today was a good day, then tomorrow is bound to be bad. If we experience success and then have something negative happen to us (and who hasn't?) we may learn that good is followed by bad.

Often, success is rewarded by giving a person more responsibility. It may feel good at first, but later it becomes a burden. Success comes frequently at the cost of things that are quite valuable: time, position, freedom and privacy. Spouses of successful people sometimes feel the price of success is the loss of time and intimacy as a couple. Subtle family messages, such as, "You can never outdo your parent," block access to our own creativity. Parents are often jealous of their children's success, good looks, intellect, gifts, grades and body image. Dysfunctional families can very subtly give messages to their children such as, "You have more than I had at your age. I had it harder than you. You had more opportunities than I did. You are getting too big for your britches."

Successful people may be defectors from a social class. Someone from "the other side of the tracks" who moves up the social ladder may become the family outcast because they have stepped over the unspoken family boundaries. In truth, we limit ourselves more than our social environment does. As a wise person once observed, "I have more trouble with me than anyone else I've ever met."

## The Fear Of Addiction
* * * * * * *

The press likes to sensationalize successful people who fail. The message is "Beware of success because you will come under scrutiny." Folklore in every culture depicts the "fool" who becomes hooked on something as a part of aging, success or getting happy and having too much fun. The list of resources which discuss the issue of human addiction and offer help in ridding us of our more harmful vices is endless. Addiction itself is one of the most severe symptoms of the "addiction-to-the-fear-of-scarcity" syndrome. We have a strong tendency to cope with fear and need by becoming addicted to substances, sex or abusive behavior.

Addiction and all of the other fears discussed in this chapter are irrational and rooted in our own decisions and attitudes. They can be changed through the concerted conscious effort and cooperation of all our inner abilities. Our minds, like our bodies, tend to become more limber, flexible and efficient with exercise.

Families involved with the processes of addiction and recovery can benefit from learning about stewardship. Some people think "stewardship" is a preachy word that only applies in a religious environment. Yet stewardship needs to become a household word because it means being responsible for what is entrusted to you by life itself. It implies action. Taking care of business, respecting others as well as yourself and being pro-active in life are all a part of affirmative self-action. Stewardship is one of the best antidotes for the fear of addiction.

## When Enough Is Enough
* * * * * * *

The day you put your foot down, throw up your hands and shout, "Enough is enough," is a wonderful day. You've reached the limits of limiting yourself. The energy you liberate when you refuse to put up with an unpleasant situation is exactly the energy you need to take positive steps. A little anger can be constructive.

# 3 Claim The Power Within

## *The First Step To Personal Power*

When you begin your journey of self-empowerment, you must first claim the force and energy that is intrinsically yours. Each of us has a built-in "power base" from which our life developed and continues to grow. In the chakra system, the first chakra is called the *Muladhara,* which means *foundation* in Sanskrit. It is located at the base of the spine, beneath the small bones of the coccyx. This chakra is believed to be the center of energy which transmits the life principle through our bodies, minds and spirits, and has existed since before we were born. This foundational chakra governs our basic raw energy, our will to survive.

Some of our most basic emotions, like passion and rage, are associated with this chakra. It is red in color. When we "see red," we are experiencing the power of the first chakra, though not its most constructive aspect.

When we reflect on the meaning of a personal power base, we need to remember that our belief systems are primary to our thoughts, feelings and actions, and are considered part of this first step to empowerment. Before action comes the idea, or the word. In the Bible the first words of the Gospel of John are, "In the beginning was the word . . ." The beginning was God who brought forth the idea of Christ before Christ came to earth.

To bring about change, we must examine our foundational beliefs and energy levels. When we reach our core issues, most of us find we have devoted much of our energy to perpetuating erroneous beliefs. If our unconscious core belief is, "I'll never get anywhere in life," an enormous amount of energy is used to keep that negative belief from reaching our conscious minds and to perpetuate it in our actions. The most important thing I can tell you is:

*Whatever you believe to be true about life*
*is exactly what you are consciously and unconsciously*
*striving to make come true for yourself during this*
*lifetime.*

## We Get Set In Our Ways And Believe
## What We Want To Believe
* * * * * * *

Most of us are under the impression that we want the best for ourselves. The problem is we may unconsciously lay our life foundations on rigid beliefs or on shifting sands of suggestion and programming from outside. In many ways we are like computers, self-programmed or designed by our families and societies to see and hear in a prescribed way. Data we take in from the environment eventually may go unnoticed. Familiar odors, sights and sounds don't affect us when we are exposed to them constantly. After a while the people living downwind of a paper mill really don't notice the terrible smell. Los Angeles natives smile and say, "Nice day, isn't it," unaware that smog is sending tears from their burning eyes. The immediate environment fades into the background as our sensory perceptions weaken. We live in our heads, but our brains numb out to routine data when it becomes too familiar.

Influencing other people to change is an extremely difficult thing to do. A friend of mine is a trainer for a pharmaceutical company. He once agreed to do some training for a rival corporation. I asked him if he thought he might adversely affect his own company's business by giving away training secrets to the competitor. He told me that such a small percentage of salesmen actually use the information he gave them, he was sure training the competition would have no measurable effect on his business.

Let's look at another example. In a classic psychological experiment, a speaker was introduced to several classes in exactly the same way, except in some of the introductions the word "cold" was included. The speaker received praise from all except those who heard the introduction using the word "cold." These students responded exactly the way they were programmed to respond.

Once our mental computers are programmed, we tend to respond to the program rather than to actual events in our lives. In this state we habitually go through the motions instead of living consciously in the moment.

## Staking Your Claim On Life
* * * * * * *

In Oklahoma we talk about staking claims. The state was settled by homesteaders who hitched up their wagons and rushed in at legally organized runs started with pistol shots. It is known as the "Sooner State" because so many settlers jumped the gun and staked their claims sooner than the official runs. The Sooners literally drove stakes into the ground to mark their territory.

I use this story to demonstrate how we make change in our lives. The settlers responded to an opportunity to get their lives grounded in reality. They used their will to make constructive change and put their lives on a firm foundation. The settlers' using the "hitching-up-the-horses" energy is an excellent example of putting our first-chakra powers to work.

The essence of change is will. When we make it come alive in our lives, our will becomes us. That decision to stake our claim in life becomes reality first by an act of will.

This doesn't mean we should strong-arm our way through life. In fact, our attitude toward claiming power has a great deal to do with healing. We can only begin to heal when we claim our healing. We *must* say that prayer, make a phone call, go out the door, get involved with asking and claiming.

If we have a difficult time claiming our power, we find a healer who acts as a sort of psychic ombudsman for us. The healer represents the seeker to himself to help him claim his will, until his "I can't" becomes an "I will." A professional healer, a psychologist for example, works with a client's self-concept and self-esteem and holds up the possibility of greater good. In 12-Step meetings, we often hear members take on the healer role by support-ing one another's claim to taking power over their lives. "We'll love you until you can love yourself," is a common phrase. A minister or rabbi or other spiritual healer will pray on your behalf and help you claim God's will for your well-being.

## Helpful Attitudes To Develop
\* \* \* \* \* \* \*

My grandfather and great uncle were both horse traders and spiritual healers. They had an unusual way of integrating the two different vocations, and I must admit that the gifts that helped them in one profession would often spill over into the other. I remember their drawing the comparison between how people treat their animals and how they must really feel inside about themselves. They cautioned me never to buy livestock from anyone who was cruel to any of their beasts or family members. These old horse traders were aware that people's own self-concepts somehow get projected onto others. In fact, people can never really separate how they treat others and how they perceive themselves. The two are deeply entwined and form a feedback loop that continually interacts.

In my years of clinical practice, I've seen the truth of this down-home observation time after time, especially when it comes to the way we treat children. We treat them the way we treat our inner child — generally the child in our life who needs the most nurturing.

## Fine Tuning Your Consciousness
\* \* \* \* \* \* \*

Taking power over your life means becoming responsible for yourself. It's about understanding and discipline. Responsibility and privilege always go together. If we are to embrace a lofty purpose or mission, we need to hold ourselves in as high regard as we hold a beautiful, high-performance sports car. We need to nourish ourselves and return to good physical, psychological and spiritual health. The beginnings of change may start on the physical level with improved diet, vitamins, weight loss or a membership at the local health club. Certainly a healthy body is part of a strong personal foundation.

An added benefit of nourishing yourself is that you tend to treat others better as well. Any significant thing that happens to us affects the way we relate to others, especially those closest to us. If we mistreat ourselves, those around us will be mistreated, too, and may rebel against us. We may not intend to hurt them, but they get hurt anyway. Children of alcoholics, for example, may not have been intentionally hurt by their parent, but they certainly suffer because of the alcoholic's self-abusive tendencies. Understanding this concept helps keep our emotional lives in balance and makes it easier for us to reach our goals.

## Good Intentions Count
★ ★ ★ ★ ★ ★ ★

Clients often say they have a more difficult time dealing with themselves than with anyone else. This means they have at least an awareness of self and an understanding of motives and intentions. Good intentions count. One of Mohammed's first laws is, "Heaven always judges us by our intentions." Making a list of your good intentions is productive when you are seeking to create new opportunities for yourself. It helps you understand your highest meaning and purpose, one that suits your true gifts and talents. You can't bring the vision to life until you have it clearly in focus in your mind.

One's true purpose *always* involves service to others. When you help others, a purpose evolves. Grace is a reward for faith. If you have faith and the will to discipline yourself to *start*, grace, or an unseen hand or spiritual presence, comes to you when you need it. Many people accomplish things they have no idea how to do. A friend had never written a book, but she was a good writer and "just knew" she could. She was not satisfied with books on creativity available for children and felt compelled to promote more authentic creativity for youngsters. When she started, she had no idea how to finish the project, but it came to her as she went along. Her first publication sold 250,000 copies. She applied her real talent for writing, her "I will" energy to serve others and believed she would get a good result. This is an excellent example of stewardship. Being a good steward of one's talents and abilities means using them in the service of others. Using your talent is the way to develop it.

## Problems Create Opportunities To Grow
* * * * * * *

In normal adult development, we grow *through* change. Some changes are predictable and should be anticipated. Other stresses appear without warning. We all have times when we feel stuck and confused, seemingly standing in mud up to our knees with no idea of how to get out of the mire. At these times of stress and confusion, we often find our creative processes energized.

Stress is the mother of all creativity; confusion can ignite our go power. A stressed-out state is one of high potential for learning. If we learn to access our inner resources, there is no need to panic. Never underestimate the positive potential of confusion — it throws us into reshifting our understanding.

In therapy if a client needs to understand a critical point, I sometimes use a technique developed by the late Milton Erickson to purposely confuse them, then give them the information they need to get out of their confusion. We don't like confusion and will latch on to anything to bring ourselves back.

## Create Fresh Options For New Problems
* * * * * * *

Do we have to create fresh solutions for every problem? Can't we rely on past experience to help us through our confusion? While past experience is never lost, we may rely on it too much. There are times when doing what worked in the past is exactly the *wrong* thing to do. If we keep on consciously or unconsciously using the survival strategies in later life that we used when we were young, we may get terrible results. As we grow and develop, we need to develop different problem-solving techniques. Clinging to old strategies can be disastrous in mid-life. Sometimes it is a matter of knowing the difference between normal and abnormal confusion.

Each situation we encounter requires fresh thought. Asking yourself the right questions can help. Ask yourself:

Is this situation exactly like the one in the past?
Am I the same as I was then?
Are circumstances the same?

If you bring attention to your first chakra while you ask yourself such questions, you may discover new options. Attention is energy. Energizing our center of will and belief can help clear our minds.

When I work with schizophrenics who are extremely confused, I take them outside and, if I possibly can, have them walk on the earth with bare feet. This grounding exercise helps clear their minds and bring them into the reality of the moment.

## Predictable Problems
* * * * * * *

In 1985 I went with more than 100 colleagues to the Carl Jung Institute in Zurich, Switzerland. We were concerned about what was happening to so many middle-aged professionals. Why was it that our group suffered extremely high rates of divorce, depression, confusion, bankruptcy and a general lack of direction in our lives?

We reached the conclusion that these situations are predictable at certain times of life, whether you are a professional helper or not. Our expectations were unrealistic. Our academic degrees did not make us immune to the realities of life. In fact, they simply made us feel worse. Our confused beliefs about how things should be were as troublesome as the natural changes that come in mid-life. We needed to find new opportunities, new choices for fulfillment, rather than clinging to stale concepts of a fairy-tale existence. For psychologists and other helping professionals as much as for our clients, claiming our healing is the way to begin creating new options.

## Creative Solutions
* * * * * * *

When we get stuck inside ourselves, our ability to see our options and create new opportunities for ourselves diminishes. Like psychologists, we become very astute at observing our own behavior. But the shift to an action mode needs to take place so that our future can begin. Our choice to believe and act establishes the foundation for tomorrow.

In 1958 Ray Bradbury wrote *The Martian Chronicles* in a weekend because he badly needed the $750 his publisher promised him when it was finished. The book is an all-time favorite. Bradbury's concepts of how it might be on Mars has shaped the world's notions of space, space creatures and beings from other planets.

Bradbury reports having a dual awareness when he wrote the book. He tells of sitting down and drawing on all the imagination and wonder he could muster, working to pull together this classic tale.

"There are actually two of me — the one who writes and the one who watches," he said later on a television interview show. "I could hardly wait to see how the book was going to end because I had no idea. I was identifying with the watcher at the time, rather than the writer."

# The Uses Of Passion

\* \* \* \* \* \* \*

Actually the doer part of Bradbury was engaged as fully as the watcher. He took the first step inside and claimed his power *to do*. It is the responsible part available to all of us — the part that claims there is a novel (or invention or job or relationship) in there — and comes up with the passion to accomplish the mission. The power of the first chakra is the power of passion, a kind of ferocity to initiate and complete things, a drive that carries us through.

Well-known interviewer Larry King says he prefers to interview people who have a chip on their shoulder. He knows they have a passion for their subject, and passion makes for a good interview.

Becoming competent and able to accept and cope with changes that occur in our lives hinges on our power to see life as it is, take a stand and make decisions. What can we expect from ourselves? Looking at the past gives us an opportunity to assess where we are now and where we want to be in the future. When we change our environment within, we create opportunities for change in our external surroundings.

"A journey of a thousand miles begins with but a single step," is a bit of Chinese wisdom, but it's important that the one step be in the right direction. The step that charts the course should be a step inside, a step toward self-responsibility and self-love. When we love and nurture ourselves and take authority over our actions, we treat all of our fellow creatures with kindness, respect and caring. We can make a difference in our world.

The Hindu Vedas suggest making one small sacrifice each day to make our goals manifest. The step can be as small as taking a minute to have a hope, a wish or a prayer. From such beliefs reality is created.

# Meditation For Life Force

This meditation reinforces our mental and emotional will. It helps us gently draw up earth energy to strengthen our life force. We bring energy through our entire body to higher levels of function and use in our lives. Repeated practice helps strengthen and bless our intention of using our will and other personal resources for good.

*Claim:* I am responsible for my own life. I can make things happen. I have a will and I am using it to improve my life.

*Affirm:* I am making my inner environment perfect through meditation. It is becoming impervious to all adverse influences and I am strengthened.

*Read:* "Seek ye first the Kingdom of God and his righteousness and all these things shall be added unto you" (Matthew 6:33).

*Meditation:* First, get grounded. Take off your shoes so you can feel the earth or floor with your feet. Sit in a comfortable position with your spine straight and your weight equally distributed on both feet. Keep your heels down and dig your toes into the floor. Feel energy coming into the soles of your feet from the earth.

Close your eyes, take a few deep breaths. Imagine that your breath is reaching the base of your spine. Visualize bright red light emanating from your first chakra, spreading through your pelvis and legs. It blends with a beam of cool pink light moving from the earth, up through your feet, up through your body and out the top of your head.

When your breathing becomes deep and regular, let your eyes roll up into your head and repeat, "The earth is the Lord's and all of its fullness is coming into me. I can build on God's foundation."

Repeat this for three minutes to the rhythm of your breath, four counts inhaled and eight counts exhaled. Pay attention to the earth energy moving up through your body, strengthening you, especially in your legs, hips and pelvis.

CHAPTER

# 4 Create What You Need

## The Second Step To Personal Power

The spiritual power of creativity is mighty. When Jesus performed miracles, he created new conditions in his followers' lives. In the gospel of John he told us we could also access God's creative power: "He that believes in me, the works that I do shall he do also; and greater works than these shall he do."

In the chakra system, the second chakra is associated with all aspects of creativity: sexuality, generativity and reproduction. Called *Svadhisthana* or *dwelling place of the Self*, it is located in the lower back at the level of the sacrum. The Self is thought to be the place of creation or chaos, where ideas are produced and the excitement of creation is experienced. This center affects the reproductive glands, the sources of procreation. The desire associated with second-chakra energy is to create, fantasize and play. Games, sports and sex are attributed to it and orange is its color. Orange is a holy color for many sects of Hindu and Buddhist monks.

Imagination is the function of mind the second chakra represents. Imagination creates desire — and desire can create destiny. This power of the mind must be understood and carefully managed. Sometimes our desires are fulfilled when we no longer really want what we've created. Desires set up in childhood may produce fruit years later. A woman friend reports longing for a daddy when she was a child but when she finally attracted the daddy of her dreams after she was a grown and competent woman in her 40s, she experienced conflict and unhappiness. She felt an extraordinary love and attraction to the authoritative man who wooed her, but by then she really needed a man who understood how to be a partner.

We can create what we need . . . and also what we don't need. The old Buddhist adage applies: *Be careful what you wish for, you may get it.* When we use the energy of this center with finesse and awareness, we create what we need to cope better with the environment. We gain access to a great deal of creative energy by understanding how to direct this second chakra potential with the complete cooperation of our conscious and unconscious minds.

## Mind Dynamics
* * * * * * *

We all have two levels of mind which are in constant communication and interaction with each other. Our conscious mind stays in the present and is in constant awareness of the here and now. This part of us thinks and guides our actions in making minute-by-minute decisions.

The conscious mind is the reality testing part that combines outside data with internal thoughts and feelings to form a plan of action.

Many theorists believe our actions are really directed by the unconscious, the mastermind of us all. It has several different layers, all of which have their own ideas about how things should be. The unconscious mind is not reality-oriented and depends on the conscious mind to interpret reality. Most creative impulses come from this level of awareness. Everyone has at one time or another found that the conscious mind somehow gets over-ridden by impulses from the unconscious. We notice it with a slip of the tongue, a clever pun or a creative insight that seems to come from out of the blue.

The communication between these two levels of mind is extremely important. The better the communication and cooperation between the different parts of your mind, the more access you have to your reservoir of resources and creative energy.

## Creating Reality With Words
* * * * * * *

The most wonderful attribute of your unconscious mind is its willingness to cooperate with you. Your unconscious will do nearly anything to help you if you know how to ask. If I say to you right now, "Don't think of a pink elephant . . ." what happens? Chances are you automatically think of a pink elephant. Your creative energy generates the mental image on cue.

Try again. Now, "Don't think of the color green." What happened again?

What this demonstrates is: *Your unconscious mind hears only the positive part of any message.* The unconscious mind does not hear *Not, Don't, Can't, Won't, Shouldn't, Weren't, Haven't,* etc. It hears no negatives at all.

*The unconscious takes the positive part of any message and feeds that information to the conscious to act upon.*

What happens when we use negatives or words ending in "not"? We get exactly the opposite of what we ask for. Imagine getting up in the morning and saying to yourself, "I hope this is not going to be one of those days" or "I hope I'm not coming down with the flu" or "Today I'm not going to smoke." What you are actually doing is asking your cooperative unconscious mind to help you have one of those days, get the flu or smoke.

## Amaze Your Family, Friends And Self
### * * * * * * *

The second step to self-empowerment entails training and using your creative ability in a constructive way.

Begin training yourself to speak and think without using negatives. Whenever you talk using negatives, you automatically set up a conflict between your conscious and unconscious mind. Our conscious mind hears "not" and our unconscious mind hears the positive part of the message and a paralyzing tug-of-war begins. How can we get anywhere when we are working against ourselves? This idea has deep and far-reaching implications in dealing with others and ourselves.

When I started my practice 20 years ago, I tested how speaking in positive language would affect patient cooperation. I always knew really good therapists helped clients understand what they *could do*, instead of what they could not do. Positive suggestions produced significant results with children. They became much more cooperative when told or asked to do something, instead of being told or asked *not* to do something.

Friends and clients began to tell me I had changed in a positive way — that I was a better person somehow — yet they were unable to put a finger on what had changed about me. When I saw my patients improving in less time than expected, I decided to try it on myself. This process is very different from the Pollyanna-ish notion of never having a negative thought. I don't believe that works. At any rate, that's a totally different method. All I was doing was talking without using negatives.

I began asking myself for help in all kinds of ways: to learn faster, retain more, to enjoy things and people more. I even began asking for help in solving problems. I applied the principle of speaking to myself in a positive way to every aspect of my life and work — things like developing better research models and doing more significant dream work to cope better with stress. Everything immediately began working better and does to this day. This simple idea has transformed people, opened doors that were closed to them and created opportunities out of the ashes of their lives.

To be more creative, begin using positive speech. Ask yourself and others what you want instead of what you don't want. Start saying and asking for things in positive language. It may seem awkward at first but amazingly your thinking, seeing, hearing and feeling take on a new perspective very quickly.

## No Buts!
\* \* \* \* \* \* \*

Using "and" in place of "but" will also add to your power to create advantageous results. The word "but" has a hidden intent — forget everything in front of the "but," here comes the real message! For example, "I really like you, but . . ." "You have been doing a good job but . . ."

"But" *can always* be replaced by "and." Say, "I really like you and . . ." or "You have been doing a good job and . . ." Use "and" instead of "but" along with positive speech when you want to give yourself or someone else a straight message and help their conscious and unconscious minds cooperate with your request. Do this if you really want them to understand fully and bring all their resources together to address a problem.

# Moving From Chaos To Creativity
* * * * * * *

There has been more philosophical and scientific change in the last 60 years than in all the centuries from the beginning of recorded history to the early nineteenth century. Change is now a normal way of life. When Alvin Toffler originated the rather unnerving concept of *Future Shock* in 1970, he was unaware how abruptly we would be thrown into that world of "things to come." Future shock, however, is no longer just one author's uncertain vision. It has become our everyday reality. We need to find creative solutions to all of life's problems.

In Genesis we find the phrase, "In the beginning God created . . ." Certainly the Bible elevates creative power to something in the realm of holy endeavor. In God's effort to make us in His likeness, He gave us the ability to create and to be creative, even if on a lesser scale. Being able to survive by generating our own creative energy is a gift God gave us when he created us in his image.

Creation is said to be the mind's best work, its finest effort. It gives body or form to an idea. However, creative solutions almost always come from chaos. Research on intelligence indicates that any great idea takes approximately 10 years to develop. When we think of the creativity of a well-known genius, we do ourselves a disservice by comparing our initial effort to his or her final results. We usually come out thinking that we lack the ability to approach, in any meager way, the important work of some of the world's greatest thinkers and inventors.

# The Creative Spirit
* * * * * * *

Let's look at the nature of the creative spirit within us to see how that energy is manifested in the things that we accomplish. Creative thought amounts to our ability *to play*. Nearly 90 percent of all six-year-olds consider themselves to be creative in some way. If we ask a young child to draw something, he will be satisfied with his picture. It is only as he grows older that he will begin to say things like, "I can't draw very well," or "I don't draw houses or people very well."

Only a very small percentage of average 40-year-olds say they have much creative ability. Social scientists have been working to find out how we lose our ability to be creative as we grow older. We know part of it involves losing our ability to play, losing our playful attitude. The ability to play, to alter reality is very closely related to our creative thought processes. Creativity is as much a playful spiritual experience as it is hard work. As adults, we restrict ourselves from gaining access to our creative energy by discarding our playfulness and combining that loss with a fear of making mistakes.

Whenever a person is hailed as being highly creative and has made many creative contributions in life, a similar scenario occurs. It is ironic that we are not usually told of the great number of mistakes they make. But, in truth, false starts become the tool with which they hone the creative process and allow it to continue to evolve.

I once consulted for a major oil company whose management team was concerned about one of its departments. This division had been recognized for its creative results but during the preceding year had lost much of its former originality.

When I met with the professionals in this division, I found they had no room or tolerance for human error. After some discussion, we discovered the root cause of the creative slump. The new department manager admitted that he valued reliable performance above originality and risk. He had systematically instilled fear in all his supervisors and employees. Mistakes were not allowed. Their fear prevented the staff members from seeking new approaches to problems.

As people grew rigid and tried to get things done perfectly the first time, they became less original and relied on old solutions. Only after they were encouraged to experiment boldly did their former energy return. Fear had frozen them into doing their work by rote. Fearlessness loosened them up again.

Mistakes are unquestionably the mark of humanity in any endeavor. Learning from mistakes eventually provides a clear path to the creative solution. Thomas Edison found more than 800 ways *not* to make a light bulb, but he had to accept the anxiety of those failures and mistakes before he reached the creative solution that would eventually bring light to the world.

## Creation And Re-creation
★ ★ ★ ★ ★ ★ ★

To live creatively involves finding ways to stop ourselves before we overdo and become overwhelmed. When stressed significantly, we may become afraid to risk and our ability to find fresh solutions diminishes. A certain amount of pressure can help creativity blossom, though there is a balance point we need to find for ourselves between having enough pressure to motivate us and too much pressure which may cause us to freeze up. Feeling stuck is a good indicator of pressure. When solutions don't come to our minds, a walk or talk with a friend, a prayer, a song or a fast game of tennis can break the pressure pattern and help our creative juices flow once again. Those who will not allow themselves to play or to dream are in serious jeopardy of losing their creative spark.

A few years ago, a large business supply firm besieged by managerial problems called me in. I quickly discovered that the managers of the company considered their most important resources the account ledgers and real property assets. I had to convince them that:

1. Their greatest resource was the potential creativity of their employees.
2. The current company policies squelched that resource.

Only then could we begin to solve problems brought about by lack of creativity.

## The Creative Needs
\* \* \* \* \* \* \*

Creativity requires the ability to adapt, to change and to some extent, the ability to survive. It particularly needs the right to fail. In order to be able to envision or perceive a situation differently from anyone else, creative people need permission from themselves and their supervisors to play with reality, to see the world in a new way and to allow access to their own fantasy.

Insane people automatically manipulate reality in their minds. Creative people do the same thing through a conscious effort. They take pride in their creations, which are an expression of their individuality. They sometimes describe the creative process as similar to a religious or "peak" experience, a bridge between the human and the divine. At a fundamental level, creativity is a guide which helps us learn about our uniqueness in a very positive way.

As a psychologist I have worked in several mental health wards and have done training and staffing at many psychiatric hospitals. In every facility I've been in, there is a rehabilitative therapy program. It may be called occupational therapy, art therapy, music therapy or some combination of these terms. All of these programs are based on the same idea: We must look inside ourselves to define and then address our needs. In other words, bringing forth what is inside you will often save you. By connecting your inner sense of being to some aspect of the outside world, you can feel this sense of accomplishment that is similar to a religious experience.

I have also discovered that creating brings a new or renewed sense of control of self and environment. Those who bring an idea into manifestation feel as if they can affect reality. Bringing an idea to fruition helps us connect our internal and external lives in a balanced way. We may not be able to create or re-create the miracles of Jesus, but each one of us has a creative miracle within, a gift, a talent, a dream. Bringing the form of a bowl out of a lump of clay may start a miracle of healing in our lives.

What if your ability to create is blocked? Without too much trouble you can find the obstacles and gateways to your own creative process.

## Obstacles To Creativity
\* \* \* \* \* \* \*

The first obstacle to creativity is fatigue. When I am involved in the intimate lives and problems of others on an ongoing basis, I need more time for rest and renewal. It is quite easy to become overwhelmed by some of the seemingly small things that pile up by the end of the day or week. It is absolutely vital that as these situations grow and change, I find the time to nurture and rejuvenate myself in solitude.

Stress causes us to pull back, to not want to risk anything. This is the best time, the most important time we can ever try something new. Remember, the greater the risk, the greater the payoff. We are ready to face the blocks that stand in our way.

One of these blocks is aging. As we grow older, we commonly get less flexible in defining ourselves. We look at ourselves negatively and define ourselves by what we lack in material goods and accomplishments, rather than by what we have internally. Growing older implies a process of adding value to our lives through knowledge, through increased awareness, through development of gifts and talents. We truly can get better at many things

. . . with no limits. But many people have a skewed set of values and denigrate their abilities and accomplishments as not really being worthwhile. We fear the risk of criticism that might come from failing, so we just don't bother. Fatal acceptance sets in. We ossify and finally die, locked into old definitions of ourselves. Habit becomes reality. We think and behave in pattern. Our awareness shrinks, our perceptions are filtered through preconceived ideas. You don't have to be elderly to experience this loss of liveliness.

One of my favorite ways to illustrate how habit clouds perceptions is to ask people to accurately draw the faces of their own watches. Very few can actually reproduce them in any detail. Misconceptions and inaccuracies appear in every case as the participants attempt to recall the image they look at about 20 times a day. In one group of 350 attorneys, not one could replicate the face of his watch. (Many of them were even wearing digital watches.) Most of us have looked at our watches hundreds, perhaps thousands of times, yet we are not really familiar with them.

If we cannot clearly remember something as static as a watch, a totally predictable image, how much more do we miss in gathering information and appreciation of people who are constantly in the process of change? Habit, along with fear of criticism and failure, is an obstacle to clear memory and to creating new solutions.

I sometimes ask clients to list their three favorite bad feelings. This approach usually catches them off guard. Few of us consciously consider our bad feelings to be among our favorite feelings. These are the feelings that occur most frequently and seem to be the most powerful within us. We need to become aware of these feelings, of what triggers them.

For instance, if we have a problem with authority, we may only need to examine our childhood attempts to grow up with a stern, authoritative parent or caregiver, someone who probably gave very little consideration to the feelings of others. For us, any encounter with an authority figure can provoke feelings of fear and anxiety.

If as a child we were abused by a man with a beard, we may today still fear all men with beards. Our fear gets rekindled by these triggers. The trigger could be as simple as the sight of a beard.

The only way out of this pattern is through it. If a client comes to me with a terrible fear of men with beards, I ask them to remember the first time they felt this fear.

They need to realize that the first time they ran away from a man with a beard, perhaps someone who had abused them, it was the right decision, a rational one. Now, however, it's time for a re-evaluation.

For the person who is afraid of bearded men, I make it a point to send her to meet a man with a beard and shake hands with him, an encounter that will diffuse her fears. The next time she meets a man with a beard, she won't feel so frightened. Her "trigger" won't be as powerful as it was. Once you address these bad feelings, they lose their control over you.

Unless we address these feelings or triggers, bring creative resources to these old problems, they will continue to harm us and become a deeply embedded part of our psychological selves.

The last obstacle to creativity comes from a false knowledge and belief. Myths about the nature of creativity thrive and flourish. You have probably heard people say with great authority, "Creativity is genius," "It takes a high I.Q." or "You are either born with the ability to be creative or not." The truth is all creativity is born from knowing how to play.

We play when we distort reality, when we change our thinking patterns and wonder, "Is there a new and different way I can deal with this situation?"

People who are severely retarded, and even most primates, seem to have creative ability that embodies a playful attitude toward problem solving. Current research on

creativity and intelligence indicates that these two qualities are entirely separate. Creativity allows us to find new
solutions to the problems we face.

## Dream Lessons
* * * * * * *

My friend Eugenie is a professional writer who usually
takes her creative process for granted. She reports having
had a series of dreams which she believes revealed to her
the nature of creativity.

She was enjoying a lazy vacation. While her husband
swam for hours each day, Eugenie walked the sand of
Florida's west coast beaches, an area known for its many
seashells. She walked and thought about her relationships
and her work and fantasized plots for new stories she
might write. She was enjoying the sun and the surf, pay-
ing very little focused attention to the thousands of shells
scattered on the beach, although she watched them to
avoid hurting her feet.

One night she dreamed about the piles of shells, some
whole, some broken, all casually and chaotically strewn
about in no particular pattern. She didn't give this dream
vision much thought.

Two nights later she had another dream in which she
saw a hundred shells, all precisely lined up on an enormous checkerboard, evenly placed along straight lines. In
the dream her attention was absolutely riveted to the
order her subconscious mind had created from the chaotic
piles of shells.

"Interesting," she thought when she awoke. "That must
be how the creative process works. It creates order from
chaos." She thanked her mind for revealing its workings
to her and thought no more about it.

Two nights later she dreamed again. This time the shells
came back in luminous, gleaming clarity. They glowed
from within, with the light of pearls, and from somewhere

a pale gold radiance shone upon them. They were neither chaotic nor orderly, but were alive with energy. They danced in swirls, upward in a continuing luminous column, with colored light playing about the edge.

"It was so gorgeous, I was transfixed. I wanted it to go on forever. This was the true nature of creativity. Chaos becomes order, which becomes ethereal beauty or art if you simply let it. I couldn't start the process consciously. I could enjoy it, be with it . . . or I could disbelieve it and stop it. I felt that it was always there, that it came as a gift when I was warm and happy and relaxed."

What a wonderful lesson we can all learn from Eugenie.

Her dreams came together in just a few nights but some time passed in between. Time is a key factor in the creative process, whether it be days, weeks or even years. Finding creative solutions can sometimes take a great deal of time. So many times you may think about a problem for a number of years before one small internal spark spurs you to "immediate" action. Employers who want a highly creative business environment need to avoid penalizing employees for their mistakes. Give people lots of permission to make mistakes and realize that these mistakes are a vital part of the creative process. You can encourage yourself to work hard at learning from mistakes. As we say in Oklahoma, "Anyone who is making mistakes is at least doing something!"

Artists across the country are once again learning to trust their insights in a 12-Step program called ARTS Anonymous. The group name stands for Artists Recovering Through The Twelve Steps. Usually a group member will speak at each meeting, talking about what happened to keep them from following their creative dreams. Invariably, group members, whether dancers, potters, painters, weavers or writers, remember in astonishing detail the day, the hour, the circumstances of the moment they gave up their creative pursuits. Their frozen memories are surprisingly complete. They recall the setting, what they had on, what was said, what the dog was doing, what was cooking in the kitchen and how they felt that fateful day.

Unfailingly it is revealed that they were stopped by criticism from someone whose opinion they valued — a parent, teacher or significant friend told them they were wasting their time, lacked talent, could never make a living with their art. Their pain is deep and hauntingly real. The support they get from each other makes a real difference in their lives.

## How To Overcome Creative Blocks
\* \* \* \* \* \* \*

If your creativity was shut down by distressing circumstances, you can take action. There are support groups you can attend, classes to join, speakers to listen to. The action of doing something as simple as singing in the church choir can bring forth your ability to become creative in other areas of your life.

Begin to empower yourself by using my steps:

1. *Energize your will.* Claim your right to be creative. Apply the go power of the first chakra to this problem.
2. *Create what you need.* Call friends, call a community center or college, look in the phone book to find a group or a class to attend. Give yourself the privilege of making mistakes. Have fun. Pursue many things before you decide which one you like best. Get enough rest. Laugh. Loosen up. Lighten up.

### Self-Evaluation

Do you feel empowered? Do you really know whether you are living up to your creative potential? Here are some questions to help you in your self-evaluation. Think about them and then write down your answers.

1. Are you really willing to accept your own mistakes? Do you have the courage to move past the need to

be right most of the time and live with the ambiguity of knowing that you do not know what to do or how to do it?

2. Can you generate a playful attitude? Are you able to fall in love with your problems? Or are your problems something that you must avoid at almost any cost? Do you accept problems as a normal part of life?

3. Do you have the perspective of a child in seeing a situation? Can you step into a child's mind or see with a child's eye the wonderment or scariness of a situation, perhaps gaining new insights from that childlike perspective?

4. Are you afraid to ask questions? If so, in what type of situations?

5. Do you have the habit of meditating on questions, thinking about them and then taking them to bed with you as a way of dealing with them?

6. Do you keep a card file of your ideas? Do you make an effort to write things down as you think of them? [I keep a running database of ideas on my computer at home, things that may prove useful later.]

7. Are you a curious person constantly exploring different ideas or are you a victim of habit addicted to a stagnant way of thinking?

8. Do you have some "holy time" for yourself, ideally in a location that is somehow sacred or new to you?

9. Are you able to feel that joining of the human and the Divine by experiencing and responding to surges of creativity? Have you done it often?

10. Do you like to try new restaurants and vacation spots or do you keep going back to familiar places?

11. When I consider all the information that comes at us daily, I am reminded of how my grandmother used to do laundry in her big tin tub. Given enough time and water, the soapsuds would work their

magic. Do you let your ideas "soak" in the very same way as grandma's laundry?

Given time, we gather more data which frequently results in a new arrangement of ideas. Remember, it takes a great deal of faith and trust in your own process to be able to create. It takes a willingness to risk and to put yourself and your ideas on the line, the way all great inventors and thinkers have in the past. Mainly it takes an attitude of unwavering confidence in yourself. You must truly know in your heart that you have tremendous resources and intuitive understanding. You feel alive because you have created, whether it's an idea, solution or a work of art.

Before you seek solutions or solve any problems, make a pact with yourself, an affirmation that you indeed are creative and have the ability to shape your own destiny. Lois Robbins, author of *Waking Up In the Age of Creativity*, writes:

> Whatever creativity is, it always carries with it a powerful sense of the mind working at the peak of its ability. Creativity is the mind's best work, its finest effort. We may never know exactly how the brain does it, but we can feel that it is exactly what the brain was meant to do.

Because action is another vital ingredient in the creative process, I offer these exercises to help you activate your creativity to analyze your personal goals. We have already discussed goal setting and its importance. Now let's begin to tap into your creative current.

## Quick Lifetime Goal Analysis
★ ★ ★ ★ ★ ★ ★

1: In two minutes write down as quickly as you can your lifetime goals with regard to personal, family, social, career/financial and spiritual areas. This is a "wish list," so write as many as you can.

**2**: In two minutes write down as quickly as you can how you would like to spend the next two years of your life. Let your imagination have full play here.

**3**: In two minutes write down as quickly as you can what you would do in the next three years if you knew that you were going to completely change your life within three months.

**4**: Select one item from each list that you feel is most important to begin working on immediately. With these three items in mind, provide problems which can only be solved with both your conscious and unconscious mind.

Remember that any goal involves thinking, writing it down, formulating a plan to achieve that goal and carrying out that plan of action. Being able to determine your goals, focus on them in written form and have an optional plan to achieve them will give you a sense of control over your life and power over your own destiny.

# Creative Energy Meditation

This meditation awakens and strengthens our generative, creative and sexual energy. It helps us move this energy to higher levels of functioning and expression. When this energy is combined with spiritually directed will, we easily control our thoughts and behavior. Creativity can be directed to our highest good.

*Claim:* I have the energy to create good in my life.

*Affirm:* Today I will seek God's vitality in the sun, bathing my body in its light to appreciate the life-giving, disease-destroying gift of the ultraviolet rays from the Lord. My body is made of light, my cells are spirit, for Spirit; they are immortal, for life.

*Read:* "And he spake many things unto them in parables, saying, behold, a sower went forth to sow; and when he sowed, some seeds fell by the wayside, and the fowls came and devoured them up: some fell upon stony places, where they had not much earth; and forthwith they sprung up, because they had no deepness of earth; and when the sun was up, they were scorched; and because they had no root, they withered away. And some fell among thorns; and the thorns sprang up and choked them. But others fell into good ground, and brought forth fruit, some a hundredfold, some sixtyfold, some thirtyfold. Who hath ears to hear, let him hear" (Matthew 13:1-9).

*Meditation:* While sitting or lying down, make yourself comfortable. Relax and begin breathing deeply. Become as relaxed as you can to accomplish a state of meditation.

The second chakra is responsible for your sexual, creative energy. Acknowledge that you are a sexual being with sexual feelings. This chakra is located at the sacral area. Visualize a radiating orange light emanating from below the navel, moving up the entire length of your body. The lower abdomen is being healed. Direct the light to surround and to gently remove any pain or discomfort from this area. See it merging with the brilliant red light from the first chakra and expanding over your entire being, melting away feelings of tension anywhere in your body. Notice any sensation or feelings that come from your abdominal area and accept them.

Repeat the following in cadence with your breath: "I can create what I need through God who strengthens me." Repeat this to the rhythm of four counts inhaled and eight counts exhaled. Do this for at least three minutes and pay attention to any sensations that arise.

# 5 Cultivate Emotional Balance

## *The Third Step To Personal Power*

Keeping the powerful energy of the emotions in balance is a pivotal point for our success or failure. We could exchange stories all day about high-level professionals who lost everything because they could not keep their conscious or unconscious emotions in check. Their desire for the good life became overblown and turned into greed or the compulsive search for instant gratification.

Many people have made it — and lost it — because their need for ego gratification outweighed their common sense with regard to business or relationships. Although if you *are* one of those people, it is very hard to discern the effect of your own negative emotions. To be able to use the power of our emotions in a consistently constructive way we need to cultivate self-knowledge, discrimination and refinement of emotional energy.

The third step to personal power involves balancing our emotional energy. It correlates with the third chakra, or *Manipura*, the seat of emotional energy known as *the city of gems*, located at the level of the solar plexus. In the process of empowering ourselves, we want to honor the positive qualities of this chakra, such as that great motivator, enthusiasm, but need to learn to control its negative aspects of anger, avarice, greed, lust and gluttony. In the most refined development of this chakra we reach a state of emotional calm. Bringing our emotional energy into alignment with our goals and purposes involves reaching a high level of integrity in which our desires are congruent with our actions.

This chakra is involved with taking in and assimilating energy from the environment and is thought to be gold in color. Its energy is particularly directed to the liver, kidney, stomach and spleen on the physical level. On a more subtle level it has to do with laying foundations for getting power over your emotions, an important life skill we should learn in adolescence, the time when this chakra is developing. Third-chakra energy helps us develop feelings — delightful in their positive form but so destructive when negative.

If your third-chakra energy is out of balance, your emotions may be disturbed enough to ruin your chances for intimacy and success. Harmonious relationships with yourself and everyone in your business and personal life can be destroyed by jealousy, pride, self-justification, self-pity, self-glorification and impatience. These negative selfish attributes are the antithesis of authentic self-esteem, which always is based on realistic assessment of one's abilities and potentials. The person with a high level of self-esteem does not need to put anyone else down in order to make himself or herself seem important.

When we develop self-knowledge it is essential to be willing to put it into action and become responsible in all areas of life.

## The Way To A Successful Life
* * * * * * *

We may have the highest intentions for establishing an intimate relationship and living a responsible life of financial independence, yet somehow we get off the track. When we look around to see what went wrong, we find a trail of compromised values and lost visions — and wonder how it happened.

Sometimes circumstances seem to go against us and we end up losing everything we have accumulated. Here in Oklahoma we experienced extraordinarily adverse economic circumstances in the last decade. When I moved to Oklahoma in the '70s, the county where I lived was one of the most prosperous in the country. In fact, it was ranked as having the third highest per capita income in any county or parish in the United States. By 1982-83 the oil-based economy had plummeted. At that point many of our friends and acquaintances were bankrupt, the suicide rate skyrocketed, the divorce rate was higher than ever before in history and all of the psychiatric hospitals in central Oklahoma were overflowing with clients.

Certainly not everyone who went bankrupt during that time was at fault, but I could see a very direct relationship between those who kept what they had and were able to recoup their losses and those who could not.

High rollers fell to the temptation to overextend themselves in high-risk investments and lavish lifestyles. When the economic crunch came, they sustained extremely high losses and could not survive financially. Some also experienced broken families and even personal breakdowns.

# The Get Rich Slow Formula

\* \* \* \* \* \* \*

An elderly Oklahoman who was quite a successful investor in stocks and bonds once gave me his secret formula for getting rich slowly.

"Son," he drawled, "all you have to do is give away 10 percent and save 10 percent of all you make. That's the secret of success for accumulating enough to maintain anyone in a decent lifestyle through old age." The Old Oklahoma Investor's 10-10 plan is a balance between personal ambition and a sense of community. He worked hard, used his gifts and talents to do the best he could and cultivated compassion and responsibility for others. Honoring his internal needs for living in harmony with his fellow human beings and his external needs for achieving a comfortable lifestyle provided him a balanced, contented life.

The Old Oklahoma Investor was a good steward. Good stewardship means making good use of what you have — your gifts, resources or tools for working your way through life. The idea of stewardship has been explored by every major religion. In the Bible, the idea of stewardship is familiar. In the Old Testament, for example, we hear of Joseph, who through God's providence helped save the ancient Israelites from starvation.

In the New Testament, the parable of the good steward tells of a rich man who needed to travel to a far country. Before he left he called his servants together. To each he gave talents, or money, according to his ability to use them. To one he gave five talents, to another two and to the third he gave one. When he returned, the servant who had received five gave him back 10, and he commended him: "Well done, my good and faithful servant. You have been faithful over a few things, I will make you ruler over many."

The person who had been given two talents gave back four, and the master commended him as well. Then the servant who had received one talent returned only one. He said he had been afraid of loss so he buried it in the ground and did not invest it. The lord was disappointed and took away the talent, gave it to the one who had 10 and cast out the unprofitable steward.

## Lessons Of Stewardship
★ ★ ★ ★ ★ ★ ★

There are many lessons for us in this wonderful story. At the time a talent was a unit of money, but the metaphor works brilliantly in translation, for we must invest our talents as wisely as we invest money. We also learn that we must use our gifts well . . . or else. If we don't, we may lose more than we bargained for. We learn that fear and irresponsibility can cost us everything. And we learn that if we are responsible and use our talents properly, we will be led to opportunities in which we will be given more. The parable tells how people handle their lives and discover how to use their gifts.

How do we reach the point of becoming poor stewards of our talents? What seems to happen is that lives get out of balance and we become vulnerable to forces and temptations we never thought were important. In the face of temptation, we run the risk of becoming selfish, greedy and vengeful.

Earlier I mentioned that one of the times you really need to be most careful is when things get too secure. That might well be the time when your footing could slip on the slippery slope of overconfidence — though it would seem to be the time you could sail smoothly through. Though there are certainly days to celebrate and relax, going to extremes and falling into a life of excess is dangerous. At all times, in good days and bad, try to maintain balance in your life.

When I speak of balance, I don't mean it as a static concept. We can't stand still in perfect balance for life would pass us by. I mean a dynamic process of staying in balance in life. There is a balance between saving and giving, between risk and security. Persons who have a natural ability to behave appropriately no matter what life deals them may have been given much affirmation or encouragement as a child. Some others may have learned balance later through trial and error, for we learn through our mistakes. Another kind of balance is achieved through forgiving and forgetting.

We have to learn to cultivate personal emotional balance, just as we must cultivate the ranch, our professions, our relationships and our investments. Our balancing act is analogous to learning to walk confidently on a ship. As we go through rough waters, it becomes more difficult but eventually we learn. In the same way, we develop an intuitive guidance system to stay in balance as we go through life. If we do not, our ship is going to start listing. The more effort it takes to right it, the more out of balance it becomes. I have often seen people ruin their health, their lives, their very beings, by not knowing how to stay in balance.

Exploring the third-chakra energy helps us find our inner balance point. In all lives that are not working well, in all cases of poor stewardship, the culprit is negative emotions. Our immediate reaction to unfavorable external circumstances may be one of fear or anger. The day the stock market takes a dive or oil prices plummet, negative emotions may drive us to act in foolish ways. If a loved one suddenly leaves or dies, we may panic and make poor decisions. Achieving emotional balance is the root of all balance in life. Use the meditation at the end of this chapter to help.

In 1945 a group of ancient papyrus manuscripts, which are now referred to as the Nag Hammadi library, were found in Egypt. The texts represent missing Gnostic (knowledge) gospels. One is the Gospel of Philip, and it is attributed to Christ and his followers. Much of its message has to do with living the balanced life. One idea I think is relevant is, "The Lord said, 'I came to make the things below like the things above, and the things outside like those inside. I came to unite them in that place.' "

This statement precisely illustrates the need for finding inner and outer balance, of becoming congruent. If you are not living in a state of congruence, your life gets out of kilter. If, for example, you believe in recycling, but you don't do it yourself, you're out of balance, not in harmony. Your inner conviction does not match your outer actions. This really suggests a lack of integrity in your life. If you believe in a Higher Power but do not honor it, you are not expressing congruency. The Nag Hammadi manuscripts also tell us that it is not possible for us to *see* the truth unless we become *like* the truth. Living according to our inner truth requires that we integrate our inner conviction with our outer actions.

Personal integrity needs cultivation. But how do we do it? Seeking that inner place of peace and calm brings us into acceptance of truth. Sometimes we are so emotionally involved with getting and keeping that we begin to think we *are* our possessions, we are our job, title, status, we are our successful husband. When we are threatened with their loss, we become furious. It's like losing ourselves. Anger can be constructive if we express it appropriately and release it in order to regain the energy that we have tied up in it. But it is very unhealthy to stay angry.

## Stress And How To Release It
**\* \* \* \* \* \* \***

I often meet adults who hang onto anger at their parents or a sibling or someone whom they feel has hurt them in the distant past. The stress this creates can hinder their spiritual and mental development for a lifetime. Stress can result from lack of forgiveness. When people say, "I will not forgive them because they are not sorry for what they did," they miss the point. You forgive another for your own well-being, not for the other person's benefit.

Revenge is inherently self-destructive too. An old Arab proverb tells us that whenever you seek revenge, you need to dig two graves. One for the person for whom the revenge is intended and one for yourself. The cost of revenge is always too high.

## Recipes For Reducing Stress
* * * * * * *

When you seek balance in your life you first come upon everyday stress. Fortunately much of it is easy to get out of the way so you can go to work on more worthy problems. By observing the following three prescriptions your ability to reduce stress is greatly improved. Virtually all of my clients have benefited from implementing these simple suggestions.

1. *Relax and pray or meditate every day.* The more you are involved in life, the more you need time to be alone and to renew yourself physically, mentally and spiritually.
2. *Get regular exercise.* Though health clubs proliferate and opportunities to work out abound, comparatively few people get regular exercise and seriously work up a sweat every day. You don't need to join a club to take a fast walk, ride a bike or jog.
3. *Eat only nutritious food.* You'll benefit from staying away from white sugar, white flour and caffeine.

## Work, Play And Relate In A Balanced Way
* * * * * * *

If you're not happy with the quality of your life and hope to find solutions, don't forget to play. I've noticed that many clients on a downhill slide neglect this important aspect of life. At work the quality and quantity of what they accomplish declines and networking ceases. In their private lives, they don't stay in touch with old friends and seem to withdraw into themselves. Depression may not be far off.

If you have a tendency to isolate, call a friend, see a movie, do something you really like to do at least one day a week. The balance point is different for each individual. Some of us truly enjoy our own company and quiet pursuits, but even if your idea of a wonderful time is reading or knitting or building models, don't overdo anything. Be a good steward of your private life, of your own happiness.

A subtle sign of imbalance is projection of feelings on others. Projection occurs when a person attributes flaws, insecurities and problems to everyone else that really describe what is going on within themselves. It is a defense mechanism we use to protect ourselves from the truth. We blame others for the very things we are experiencing, but are unwilling to admit, even to ourselves. If we begin to ascribe anger or depression to others, we may well be witnessing a reflection of our own troubled inner life.

## Emotional Stewardship For Relationships
★ ★ ★ ★ ★ ★ ★

In our marriages and other close relationships, we are prone to getting into emotional tugs of war. Getting our own way becomes more important than relating. Emotional contests of will take place in families, the workplace, on the playing fields, in organizations — in every field of human endeavor.

Certainly the idea of stewardship transfers beautifully to these relationships, having to do with "responsibility for sharing systematically and proportionately your time, talent and material possessions for the benefit of all." In other words, emphasis is placed on fostering, furthering and encouraging those you are in relationship with, not ignoring or competing with them. Enlightened business practice stresses having people work *with* you, rather than *for* you.

When we allow a marriage to deteriorate into a kind of domestic business arrangement, we are not practicing good stewardship. Good stewardship requires not only care of externals, such as the house and the car, but also requires that we cultivate the more subtle realm of feelings. Marital problems cannot be solved by a couple merely resolving problems about their children, money, home, lawn or in-laws.

## Refining Your Relationships
* * * * * * *

Everyone, from newborns to centenarians, needs appreciation. Acceptance and appreciation are such basic needs that whenever I'm called upon to help my clients resolve marriage problems, I begin by looking at their level of perceived appreciation for each other.

When a couple first gets together, the chemistry is great. You feel as if you have at last found true joy. The wonderful feeling of finding someone who you believe is entirely empathic, kind and sympathetic to your intentions is profound. The whole idea of falling in love is expressed one way or another in nearly every song, novel, TV show, movie, poem and art form. Everyone is in love with love.

When couples first couple, they have the remarkable ability to create a personal island in the midst of a sea of stress. It is amazing how they have the ability to fill each other's cup mentally, physically and even spiritually. Somehow the couple manages to get away from it all, to delve deeply into the comfort of each other's company. This magic works very well for a while, but when you examine this couple a few years later, you may well find freeways running across their island, telephone cables crisscrossing it and all of the beaches inhabited by other people.

As I look at their situation, I ask myself, What happened to their wonderful secluded island? How did they lose the ability to be intimate? To have meanful conversations with each other? Why do they behave as if they hate each other?

In counseling we first address the amount of time they spend together. I always ask each of them to look backward. How is the amount of time they spend together different from the amount of time they spent together at the beginning? The answer is always the same: They no longer spend much time together, they don't feel that their partner appreciates them. If the relationship is still alive at all, they then say they would like to spend more time together because they used to enjoy it a great deal. But there are so many demands on their time, they can't be with each other enough.

Lack of time and appreciation for each other is the root cause of couples falling out of love, getting bored with life, trading intimacy for security and settling for "level D" marriages. Living out a ho-hum marriage is a drain. You may just feel a little bored, but that may be just the tip of an enormous iceberg dragging your spirits down. Boredom is a negative emotion and it pulls the rest of your life out of balance.

## Breaking Through The Boredom
* * * * * * *

We get out of life what we are willing to settle for. To become assertive in order to get what you want from a relationship may seem threatening, but the truth is that in any relationship, especially in a marriage, you will get far less than you bargained for unless you assert your needs.

Assertion is not aggression. In close personal relationships, unbalanced emotions can lead to the level of personal attack or even physical violence. If you want your relationship to work, develop listening skills and let each person have their say for a specified period of time. Let your partner express his or her needs uninterrupted for 15 minutes, then express yours for 15 minutes. The *uninterrupted* is as important as the needs, for it indicates that someone is interested, cares how you feel and wants to know what you need. Good listening indicates appreciation. If you can't listen for 15 minutes without interrupting, that's a good indication that you need to work on your own state of emotional equilibrium. Remember, in personal negotiation there is no place for blaming, shaming or attacking in any way. It is about saying in a positive way what you want and need.

In a relationship each person has a right to their fair share of time and attention and a right to say no. Maintaining everyday life together fulfills only part of that need. But a good relationship requires both partners to contribute to creating aliveness for themselves and for each other.

Whether your primary relationship is a marriage or not, each partner has to take responsibility for keeping it fresh. Together you can negotiate the time you will spend and activities you will engage in. In the same way that you negotiate with your inner personalities, expect to give up something to get something. Remember that if you make a bargain, you must live up to it or the consequences may be dire. A marriage is a covenant in which both partners give up a certain amount of autonomy in favor of the partnership. The two of you together become an *us* and supposedly operate for the greater good of the whole rather than for individual ego satisfaction.

## Seeking Emotional Honesty
* * * * * * *

People who are very accomplished or successful are often the ones with troubled relationships. The high achievers of life are often adept at performance skills.

They put on a facade so often that eventually their true selves become obscured and they forget who they once were and really are now. When someone lives a life that is not emotionally honest, the partner suffers — particularly the partner in marriage or another close relationship. When performance becomes your life, it's hard to stay emotionally honest, even with yourself. We see this syndrome in media stars and in super salespersons, but we also see it in people like kindergarten teachers who feel they are always required to be cheerful, chipper, perky and "on." And we see a lot of it in marriages.

No sooner have couples left the altar than they begin to play what they perceive to be their designated roles of The Husband and The Wife. This is a particularly sticky wicket, for when we become husband and wife, we do vow to fulfill our responsibility to make the marriage work. But our functions need to be negotiated in advance — and open to renegotiation.

In many marriages, emotional honesty gets left in the dust as Jane and John opt for performance. Naturally they become resentful, for the marriage, which should be a freeing experience, becomes repressive.

"He doesn't love me for myself," I hear wives moan in therapy. "He just wants a servant." And husbands complain, "She just wants a paycheck."

In any relationship, particularly marriage, we tend to mold it to be whatever we subconsciously believe it will be. Often relationships turn out to be replicas of our own histories. We unconsciously marry someone who is much like our parents, and "parentize" our relationship. The pattern becomes clear when one partner becomes overly spouse-dependent. If one partner tries to force the mate into becoming a parent, then he or she is free to regress to childhood. It is very difficult to be romantically involved with an emotional child.

It's not atypical for men to "motherize" their relationship with their wives. They generally expect wives to nurture and take care of them as if they were children, but on the surface it looks just the opposite. Men are brought up to believe that they should be able to take care of women and want it to look like they do. The Lone Ranger, that paragon of machismo, never got close to anyone, but was always respectful to women and always had the last word.

One modern Lone Ranger I know had trouble driving because he had weak eyes. When they took trips together, his wife would drive hundreds of miles, then get out and let him drive the last mile home so their neighbors would think he was fulfilling his role as protector of the Little Woman. Was this a big thing? Probably not in itself, but it was an indicator of deep emotional dishonesty in the marriage. Keeping up appearances was more important to this man than relating in an honest way to the interesting, competent person his wife was. He was interesting and competent as well but saved it for the office and rarely shared that part of himself with "The Wife."

In relationships bound by role-playing, neither partner is able to play with the other or bring spiritual renewal into each other's life, even though that may have been what attracted them to each other in the beginning. Unless they can leave their roles behind and become honest about their emotions, the stage is set for pursuing extramarital affairs in an attempt to capture what has been lost. For men, especially in mid-life, an affair or even a brief liaison with a prostitute seemingly provides a moment of pseudo-intimacy, fun and excitement.

If we heed the lesson of the third chakra, however, we understand that these men are emotionally underdeveloped and have reverted to adolescent pursuits at mid-life. Clinging to immaturity is not conducive to establishing real personal power. Women make the same mistake when they take lovers outside marriage.

Some marriages need to end. Some extramarital romances turn out to be extraordinarily good relationships, but most of the time they are attempts to fill the void left by emotional dishonesty in the marriage.

Women tend to want different kinds of relationships with men. Sometimes they may make men into father images, sometimes they want to mother men, but what most women really want, I believe, is to have a spiritual covenant with a man. They envision having more freedom and friendship in their relationships than most men can fathom. They long for a you-and-me-against-the-world alliance and may even feel *called* into a relationship, hoping that covenant will give meaning to their lives. Happy marriages may result. But not necessarily.

If women give up too much of their lives in order to become the Total Woman and otherwise fulfill fantasies of men and society, they may do themselves, their partners and their children a real disservice. (A friend of mine calls them Totalled Women.) If they are not true to themselves, what kind of model are they for the boys and girls they raise? Like the kindergarten teacher who always has to be perky and cheerful, they present only a superficial understanding of humanity to their children and may actually contribute to their children's search for meaning outside of the home — a search that may lead to drugs and worse. How can children, particularly teens, learn emotional depth, compassion and honesty from parents who are giving shallow performances all the time?

Truthfulness and respect are what make relationships work. These qualities add more to our personal lives than anything else and form the foundation of all love and intimacy.

## How We Avoid Truth
* * * * * * *

There are four fairly effective ways to get away from truth. See if they ring a bell for you.

1. *Denial.* Just deny that it is real. If we don't want to see the negative, we pretend it does not exist. We reject unpleasant truths by consigning them to the dumpster of our consciousness. They don't exist and we don't have to confront them. When the town drunk says, "I am not an alcoholic," that's denial.

2. *Minimization.* We tell ourselves it's not really so bad, and anyway, it's going to get better, just you wait and see. In truth, things rarely get better without help. We can cut down all this timber because, after all, there's more over the next hill. (Not any more. We need to replant.)

3. *Distortion.* We simply tell half-truths or exaggerate things. This may be wish fulfillment or a desire to be accepted and admired by others. Our wish may be so strong, we are willing to compromise by being untruthful. Income tax forms and resumes are places we may see distortion.

4. *Lies.* Telling a boldface lie always catches up with you and hurts your relationship with whomever you lied to.

# The Problem Of Congruence
* * * * * * *

Making things below like things above, as the Gnostic gospel discusses, entails a search for meaning and purpose. What we are doing today may not reflect our deepest desires and the highest manifestation of our gifts.

If we grew up in families that exerted too much discipline and control over us, we learned to deny our deepest desires and to conform with our parents' notion of who we are, how we should look, feel and behave and what we should do with our lives. If they were strict or scornful, we may even feel guilty for wanting something different. Our true desires are buried below in our subconscious minds, while above, in our conscious lives, we present a face to the world that does not reflect our true character.

The need to find our true selves is one of the best problems life can hand us. It is always an opportunity for growth, change, success and contentment. One of our purposes is to stay vividly alive and awake to the opportunities within.

## Finding Your True Desires
* * * * * * *

Every person basically knows deep inside what they want out of life, what goals they want to accomplish and even the types of relationships they want to have. At the same time they are often unaware of their intentions at a conscious level. Psychologists often see clients who are uneasy and unfulfilled with their lot in life and wonder whether they are following their true path. After much discussion and batteries of aptitude and ability tests, they are rarely surprised at what the data reflect about their real talents and gifts. Our psychological defenses disguise our desires from us — especially lack of permission from internalized parents to have what we really want.

When a client asks, "What shall I do about this situation," I know it's time to get out the mental Windex and start cleaning the windows of perception. A new view is called for.

Once we have raised the issue, it must be addressed in a practical sense. We need to ask ourselves how to align our desires with our abilities and create opportunities to put them together in a constructive way.

If an insurance executive would rather be a forest ranger, what does he or she do? Once we have pinpointed our desires, we begin to see change take place no matter what we do. If there is really a purpose in our lives, it is to stay on the road and keep traveling. We bring the luggage of our experience with us and open it up to bring out appropriate skills and abilities that transfer to our new goals. We may also decide to go back to school, move, get new training. We open the eyes of our souls and look at life from a new perspective.

Some people believe that we were born to follow our heart's desire. We were given the desire as a gift, and it is always the best use of ourselves to follow it. Our desire is a mandate we must follow to find our true place in the scheme of things. Cultivating our desire, becoming its steward, is the only way to find contentment and fulfill our purpose. If we fail to do so, our emotional energy will always be divided and everything will be tinged with regret. The worst thing we can do to ourselves or our children is thwart that desire.

Listen when little Katy says she wants to be an actress. Foster and nurture her and take her seriously. Perhaps it is her true gift. If you discover in yourself a lust for acting when you're middle-aged, don't overlook the possibility of joining a community theatre group. Even if it's too late to become another Meryl Streep, you can still provide yourself with pleasure and a sense of accomplishment if you follow your dream.

It's hard to get parents to acknowledge it, but they may be jealous of their child's talents and stand in their path, subtly — or not so subtly — putting down their gifts. It is bewildering and painful for the child and may cost them their chance for happiness in life. Employers may wreak havoc on their employees in a similar fashion. Talented people often report getting hired for their talents and then having them diminished by a boss who is jealous. Sometimes keeping emotional balance requires some very painful self-examination to see if you may be hurting others or yourself with your negative emotions.

Ultimately our best chance for happiness hinges on finding the path that engages our positive energies and enthusiasm and would appeal to us no matter what the rewards might be. If you go into a field such as medicine or law or publishing for the rewards, you will be mediocre at best and truly miserable at worst. Being a happy carpenter is far preferable to being a miserable investment banker. The emotional cost is too great to compensate for the financial rewards.

## When Is Enough Enough?
★ ★ ★ ★ ★ ★ ★

Sometimes in our quest for self-empowerment we go too far. Books and magazines report an accelerating rate of change that almost everyone has to adapt to and keep up with — or else. But it's possible to weaken yourself and your special gifts if you push yourself too hard. They are not given to you to commit suicide with. Please don't wear yourself out trying to be superman or superwoman.

Even Mother Teresa has limits. It's not her job to save everyone in India, she has said. It's her job to be faithful to what she does. And this means taking the time to stop when necessary.

Jesus had a good sense of when enough was enough for him. Several times in his ministry he said, "Let us go to the other side of the lake," and got into the boat and went somewhere else. Why didn't he stay where he was and work all night? If you are gifted, you are vulnerable to having your gift weakened by overuse. I believe his actions tell us to be good stewards of our energy and gifts.

When you are working on something, how can you tell whether you are starting to tilt into the abusing-your-gifts column? In any situation just ask yourself:

1. Is my talent being used for the purpose it is intended?
2. Is this an appropriate time and place to use it?

If the answer to both of these is yes, you're probably all right. By asking the question, however, you're indicating you may be close to your limits.

Using the power of the third chakra can help us cultivate our talents, define our limits, keep us in emotional balance and prepare us for further growth. When we clear out old emotions and learn to understand and deal with new ones that come up, we keep the path toward tomorrow free of obstructions. The way to true opportunity, happiness and contentment in life is through refining and respecting our emotional energy. We can't just ignore it and expect to have life work.

# Meditation For Balanced Emotions

This meditation energizes our ability to soothe our emotions and keep them in balance. Repeated practice serves to promote tranquility and feelings of peace.

*Claim:* I cultivate a sense of order and balance in my life.

*Read:* "And he said, Whereunto shall we liken the kingdom of God? Or with what comparison shall we compare it? It is like a grain of mustard seed, which, when it is sown in the earth, is less than all the seeds that be in the earth. But when it is sown, it groweth up, and becometh greater than all herbs, and shooteth out great branches; so that the fowls may lodge under the shadow of it" (Mark 4:30-32).

*Meditation:* While sitting or lying down with your spine straight, take a few deep breaths, getting as relaxed as you need to accomplish a desired state of meditation. Imagine a bright yellow light that is emanating from your solar plexus area.

The third chakra is the seat of emotions. Acknowledge that you are an emotional being and that your creativity is boundless. Feel the brilliant yellow light moving outward from the middle of your stomach area throughout your body, up into and out of the top of your head. See the yellow light blending with the red and orange lights moving around your being.

Repeat the following in cadence with your breath, *"I am making my emotional environment clear by focusing only on good feelings and positive outcomes."*
Repeat this to the rhythm of four counts inhaled and eight counts exhaled. Do this for at least three minutes and pay attention to any sensations that arise.

# 6 Set Your Heart On Your Goal

## The Fourth Step To Personal Power

Once we have come to understand how the intrinsic qualities of our lower chakras — our will, creative potential and emotional energy — can be brought to awareness and put to use to help us on our journey toward self-empowerment, we reach the level of the heart energy of the fourth chakra. For most of us, committing our hearts to setting and reaching new goals may feel almost threatening. We are reluctant to risk opening our hearts because they have been broken in the past. We've learned to bury our hurts and bravely shoulder on. Once you are aware of the almost magical qualities of the heart's energy, I hope you will be encouraged to bring its full power into your life at any cost. Do everything wholeheartedly.

In the symbology of many cultures, we know the invincible power of the heart — leaders who are great-hearted or lion-hearted have courage and conviction, they never give up, never say die. In more sensitive endeavors such as art, a performance or work comes to life when it touches our hearts. The heart represents life itself.

While courage is a positive attribute of the heart, we nevertheless disempower ourselves when we shut down our more tender feelings of love and compassion. Can we persist in difficult situations without losing our humanity? General Norman Schwarzkopf, commander of allied forces in the Gulf War, is a good example of someone who used all the energy of the heart. In news broadcasts this strong man was frequently seen with tears on his face.

"I'd never trust a man who couldn't cry," he told an interviewer.

The fourth chakra lies near our heart. It is the center chakra, lying between the three lower and three upper chakras. In the same way, the qualities of the heart are central to our well-being. Called *Anhata* in Sanskrit, it means *love stricken*, and is associated with an unheard sound, an eternal note not struck by human hands. Like the other chakras, the fourth chakra represents a dynamic process — in this case, the process of loving and taking heart. The subtle energy of this chakra governs the chest and is transmitted throughout our upper bodies, affecting our arms, hands and sense of touch. It is associated with the color green, which represents healing. Opening the heart chakra allows us to reach higher levels of consciousness and ascend to a more significant plane of living. Through its energy we allow ourselves to be touched by tenderness and grace.

The fourth chakra, sometimes called *the abode of mercy*, is also the place of forgiveness. In order to completely forgive someone, we need to go beyond words and express mercy in both our words and actions. Until we can implement forgiveness in our lives, the energy of the heart is not fully available.

We all like to think of ourselves as loving, but are we? Our ability to love depends upon how good we are at forgiving, not how good we are at loving. Though some may think loving and forgiving are the same, I have found that the ability to love deeply comes from the ability to forgive deeply — first.

In all of the world's great systems of learning, the power of love is accorded the highest respect. In the Book of Proverbs in the Old Testament we are told, "Guard your heart with due diligence, for out of it come the issues of life." Christianity is based on the message of love and forgiveness taught by Jesus. He referred to love as the greatest gift of the spirit.

For many of us, the person who needs our love and forgiveness the most is ourselves. We have internalized messages of shame and blame received in childhood and continue, unconsciously, to perpetuate the errors of our parents and teachers. We may even have received erroneous messages about God and be in terrible conflict about spirituality. Perhaps you need to forgive God as well as yourself and your parents.

Many people seek therapy to recover from the wounds of the past, which may be a good idea for you. Whether you choose therapy or not, the bottom line is to become responsible for your own life. Forgiveness of yourself and others is the key to moving on.

To set your heart on change requires that you love formulating your plans and carrying them out. In a sense it means learning to cherish or love each and every one of your problems. This may seem like a superhuman task, suitable only for gods and goddesses, but I assure you, you can bring the power of love into your life and use it to persevere in reaching your goals.

# Becoming Wholehearted

**★ ★ ★ ★ ★ ★ ★**

Becoming wholehearted requires development of new awareness and willingness to move beyond the past. Setting our hearts on change is easy for anyone who is not carrying wounds of the past. But how many of us are really free from old wounds?

Old hurts lead us to try to solve our problems by blaming someone else. Settling on such an elementary form of problem-solving prevents our minds from generating creative solutions. In blaming others for our problems, we relinquish the control we have over our own lives. We are giving away our personal power.

I once had a client who began talking about how little control he had over his life the minute he came into my office. He felt that because he had no control, he had no chance of ever changing his life. I asked him to tell me how he kept himself from changing, and he replied that it was someone else's fault. I asked him to assume he would change his life in a positive way and forever. I assured him that this change would only be permanent if he had the courage to do one thing: to assume full responsibility for anything and everything that happened to him.

He needed to understand that until he was willing to absolutely stop blaming others for everything that had happened in his life, he would never be able to free himself to create more positive opportunities. Negative behavior becomes a self-fulfilling prophecy when we give control and responsibility for our lives to someone else, which is what we do when we blame them. If it's their fault, that means they did it. Such an attitude makes changing ourselves impossible.

In the Bible, the Book of Romans presents a very curious and interesting statement: "All things happen toward good for those that love the Lord." When people reach a point in their lives where they are willing to make a commitment to growth and understanding, they will make the best of any situation. Forgiving releases us from the responsibility of carrying anger and blame inside us. We are then free to make choices based on reason rather than emotion.

When we accept full responsibility for our problems, we will be able to love them and think of them as opportunities for growth. At that point, new options may automatically appear. And they may have significance beyond our wildest imaginings. History tells many tales of those who invented products, services and problem-solving techniques others found valuable when they were simply trying to solve their own problems. Many health-care professionals enter their chosen field in response to their own needs, but they help countless others along the way as they seek their personal solutions. Even members of Alcoholics Anonymous and other 12-Step groups help one another immeasurably when they just show up to maintain their own sobriety and share their personal experience, strength and hope.

Increasing numbers of adults in their 20s and 30s are unable to effectively handle crisis or conflict. Consequently, they are returning home to live with their parents instead of seeking more satisfying solutions to their dilemmas. They seem to lack the perseverance needed to see and opt for more creative alternatives in their lives. Without a sense of purpose to ground them, they remain in a twilight zone between childhood and adulthood.

Conflict can teach us much if we will only allow ourselves to learn from it. If we can keep our feeling of conflict within a range where we can tolerate working on the problem, then creative solutions can come to pass and become real object lessons in our lives.

## Renew The Heart By Facing Pain
* * * * * * *

Almost daily in my practice I listen to people who tell me about situations in which they felt emotionally annihilated. Yet, by accepting their problems instead of fighting against them, they gained strength.

Grief is one problem we must all deal with. Whenever we are confronted with a death of any kind, whether it is the loss of someone we love or the loss of something like a job, status, health or an expectation, it's natural for us to grieve. Working through the grief process brings out either the best or worst in any person. The experience of grief tends to come over us in waves and feels like standing at the beach about chest high in the breakers. We attempt to stand up yet, no matter how hard we try, we still feel like we're drowning.

If we can allow ourselves to move *with* the waves, instead of fighting them, we will feel them less intensely and less frequently. If we fight them in anger, we will quickly lose our strength. Although grief is extremely painful at times, it is our best teacher. It forces us to delve deep inside ourselves to bring forth new options for change. Most people do not want to remain in pain for very long. Experiencing grief and loss may encourage us to change and allow us to adjust realistically to our loss.

## Psychodynamics Of Change
* * * * * * *

Change is a very difficult thing for many of us to accept. In any decision involving a great deal of change, we experience conflicting emotions. It is much easier to stay where we are, to accept the status quo. Researchers found that whenever a person or animal reaches the point of change, they feel some degree of fear or anxiety. A starving wild animal will hesitate when coming upon a dish of food. You've probably heard of someone who had so much anxiety they backed out of getting married at the last minute. Some people don't go on vacations, decide not to move or take a new job simply because it involves change. The anticipation of change is too anxiety-producing for them to be able to carry through. But if we let ourselves have feelings of anxiety and persist wholeheartedly anyway, we find positive feelings increasing as we near our goal.

Once we reach that goal, our good feelings continue to grow, and our negative feelings tend to diminish or actually disappear.

Fear of change can cause us to become very negative. We feel threatened by the impending change and experience a need to proceed as quickly as possible beyond this point. This is when we need to slow down, to listen and learn from these feelings. Once we make the change, the negative feelings will almost always diminish on their own.

Could all of this internal conflict that drains our courage and robs our hearts really be necessary? Does it serve any useful purpose? Psychologists agree our personalities are comprised of many different parts. Sometimes these different personality parts are called ego states. These states are often presented to us as a parent, an adult and a child. These are not separate personalities, but simply different roles in which we experience the various aspects of our lives. In addition to being defined as the different roles we play in our lives, they can also be manifestations of different moods we experience. The more creative an individual is, the greater his capacity to hold differing ideas, thoughts and feelings about a situation at the same time. For example, someone can really like chocolate, but at the same time know that it would be unwise to eat too much of it. We can have approach/avoidance conflicts regarding places, people, things and ideas. Different parts of us experience different aspects of any situation.

Our personalities share some common structures. One is the childlike part of us, the playful part. Another is an opposite-sex set of experiences referred to as the *anima* and *animus* that sometimes comes into play in our actions and behavior. One model of loving supposes one person's "maleness" loves the "femaleness" in the second person and that the "femaleness" in the second person loves the "maleness" in the first person. The thought may arise, if I were a man I'd be you, or, if I were a woman I'd be you.

In any kind of coupling then, we have at least two kinds of relationships. At different levels, we may actually love the other person and also love our own opposite-sex part. To make relationships even more complex, the third part of our personalities is like a parent who may take very critical and then very supportive stances. Some clients have described this level of consciousness as having some kind of protector or a wise older person inside them.

There is also another part to our personality, which Carl Jung referred to as our "shadow" or "dark side." Although we may be reluctant to admit we have a dark side, it is there. We need to remember that all of our inner selves have a positive quality we can learn to nurture: They all want us to survive and stay in balance. Sometimes conflict comes about because these different parts simultaneously require different things and have different values. Conflict may lend richness to our lives and increase our options.

## Learning To Love Our Ego States
* * * * * * *

Normally all of us can see two sides of any question or problem. Often we even take the opportunity to discuss both sides, or at least listen to both sides of an issue when we are making a decision. What we are listening to are those psychological personalities or entities inside us who give us varying types of information. Often we sense negativism and pessimism from deep inside. We can learn to handle these feelings by getting all of our parts to cooperate and work together. When each part works individually, conflict comes in and drags us down, crippling our capacity to make decisions. To regain our feelings of power, we must reach an agreement among the different parts of ourselves on what course of action we shall choose.

Another aspect of our ego states that leads us away from self-love and acceptance is the tendency to put ourselves down and assume guilt for having negative thoughts. That negative cycle can continue endlessly and damage our sense of personal power.

There is a very specific program of change we can use to deal with our negative thoughts and cope with our inner conflicts. To begin this process, we must first remember that the intention of our unconscious mind is to give us protection and to keep us from being overwhelmed by responsibility. This change process allows us to reach the peak of our empowerment. Using the following steps will persuade our different levels of consciousness to work together in harmony. You can only reach this harmony when and if you are fully ready to take complete responsibility for your own life. You cannot blame others for your inability to live up to your potential as you see it.

You will be amazed at the things that you can accomplish once you master the following technique. You will know what your unconscious as well as your conscious mind is willing to do to help you. Remember, your unconscious mind will offer you limitless support in any decision or course of action. I like to refer to this seven-step technique as the Ultimate Opportunity Process. When you work through this process, your inside and outside will cooperate, work together as a goal-directed team and you will reach high levels of integrity and congruence.

This technique has proven itself to me many times over the years. One Saturday night I was returning home late from a dinner party with a carload of people. The dinner had been held at a restaurant approximately 100 miles from my home. As I began driving home, I discovered that everyone else in the car had gone to sleep and I was becoming quite sleepy too. I tried all the normal things one does to stay awake and alert. I rolled down the window, played the radio, sang to myself but nothing worked. I just kept getting sleepier. Finally, out of desperation, I decided to take action. Rather than stopping the car and asking someone else to drive, I began to communicate with my internal parts. I thanked these parts of me for letting me know I was getting sleepy. Instead of fighting them or blaming them for my problem, I sent them my wholehearted love. At the same time, I asked their help in assisting me to get home safely. I discovered that when I struck a bargain with myself, negotiating to take a nap after church the next day, I immediately became awake and alert. I reached home safely about an hour and a half later with my carload of sleeping passengers.

I had been able to communicate my needs internally and to ask for cooperation and help from my different parts in assisting and protecting myself and the others in the car. This relieved me from the overwhelming demands of staying awake, which at first I thought was impossible.

Since then I have used this technique many times, on myself and with my clients. Now you can learn to use it for yourself. Remember, this technique can only be fully utilized if we begin with a loving, blameless and forgiving perspective.

## The Ultimate Opportunity Process
* * * * * * *

1. Whenever you experience a symptom, go inside yourself and thank that part of you that is causing the symptom. Consider the symptom from a parent's point of view and then from an adult's point of view. Our symptoms can be anything that bothers us: a pain in the neck, a stomachache, headache, general fatigue or any unwanted thought. Thank your inner part for its intention of trying to help you. Although this process may sound ridiculous, what you are

actually appreciating is the concern and protection offered to you by your internal safety system.

2. Our symptoms teach us. Any symptom is a signal that we are not satisfied. Ask the part's cooperation in helping you to achieve a more satisfactory outcome for whatever it is trying to teach you. The secret here is to be very respectful of yourself since your symptom is a messenger sent to help you gain personal power.

3. Ask the part that is giving you the symptom to make a contract with you. The contract is that he, she or it will give you three things to do *right now*. If you do these things, the symptom will go away with the condition that the personality part that is giving you the symptom will never lose the power to protect you unless it desires to give up that power.

At this point, you may be wondering if we are entering the area of mysticism or hypnosis. Let me assure you that absolutely the opposite is true in this case. This program is a logically-based proven system that works if you invest the time and effort to do what I am proposing — to, literally, make an agreement with yourself. The agreement might sound like this: "I will behave in a specified manner, if all of us will come up with a mutually-agreed-upon method of behavior or a course of action to alleviate the stated problem or symptom."

4. Watch, listen and be aware of your feelings so you may receive messages that surface. Our unconscious mind communicates with us in many different ways. Sometimes a poem will come to mind, a saying, a scripture verse or perhaps a verse from a Psalm. There can also be such things as mental or visual flashes of symbols or images that in some way have a bearing upon or relate to the symptom or problem. The language of the unconscious mind is expressed

strictly in symbols. Thus what we must do to understand the message from deep inside ourselves is to understand the symbol which our minds give us.

The third way our minds communicate with us is to give us an old "feeling." It can be a feeling we once had, or a memory of an experience that has been helpful to us in solving past problems. Understanding these feelings will lead us to new ways of resolving current problems.

The fourth way our unconscious minds communicate with us is to give us ideas in terms of smell. Memories are very closely linked to our sense of smell. Sometimes, in fact, when we need to work on something, or experience dealing with a new kind of concept, we will have a flashback to former feelings which are linked to a specific aroma.

Our sense of taste works in a similar way. People often will connect experiences with tastes they associate with certain specific situations. I once worked with a young man who described people in terms of different types of food. He would automatically know if he was going to like somebody or not by the kind of food that he was reminded of.

5. Thank the inner part of you for its messages and write down or tape anything that seems to answer your question. Any hunches, thoughts, images or ideas that you get during this process are parts of the answer. Once again, be sure to thank the responding part of you for its message.

6. Go within yourself and ask all parts inside of you if there is any part that disagrees with the overall plan. (If you get a strong feeling of disagreement, go back to two and start again.)

7. As soon as you make a plan, execute it immediately. Do something positive for yourself and realize that it is okay to feel safe by yourself. Work hard if that is what the plan entails. Be positive with yourself. Re-

member to use positive language, and to let yourself speak without using the words "don't," "won't," "shouldn't," "can't" and "not." This use of positive language is necessary because the unconscious mind interprets self-language. The primary goal at this point is to formulate a plan and to allow yourself to work the plan. In this way, you are keeping the contract with yourself.

*Warning: You must understand the seriousness of this procedure. Any commitment that you make to yourself must be made in earnest.*

If you make a contract with yourself and fail to carry out that contract, it is very probable that your symptoms may increase and that it may be even more difficult to re-establish trust with yourself in making another contract. Every time you make a contract which requires taking immediate action, your symptoms will decrease and your unconscious and conscious minds will receive great learning from within. Take three separate action steps right away to reinforce your inner power. For example, write down your idea, make a phone call, check facts or figures with a printed source. The greatest lesson to learn is to become aware of the power that you have to make things happen for you. Spend as much time working on the Ultimate Opportunity Process as you need.

For this technique to be effective, you must want with all your heart to empower yourself to be all that you can be. Using the process will alleviate your symptoms, give you more power, decrease your indecision in every situation. You will feel more powerful in your interactions with other people and they will see you as being much more positive. It begins with seeing your problems as opportunities to learn about yourself and to become more efficient.

Engineers have this attitude whenever they start to design products and machines. They understand that whatever breaks down or wears out in a machine is something that needs strengthening. They view problems as opportunities. When machines are inefficient, engineers know something needs to be fixed. Breakdowns are part of the feedback system, signaling how the product or machine can be improved.

It is scary to break through your patterns of behavior and choose to do things differently. You may need to work your way through fear at the same time you maintain the direction toward positive change. If you know your mind will come up with all kinds of reasons why this situation would *not* work for you, or *why* you should keep yourself from changing, you will be prepared to handle the objections. Be aware that the closer you get to bringing about some important change, the more you may feel you need to back off and forget the whole project. We humans always prefer to "go with the devil that we know."

Seeing things differently and accepting new ideas takes a lot of courage and a strong sense of self. It takes more than just the ability to daydream. Lois Robbins, in her book, *Waking Up in the Age of Creativity*, describes the creative process in six stages:

1. Preparation
2. Frustration
3. Incubation
4. Illumination
5. Elaboration
6. Communication

We can block ourselves at any one of these stages if we see ourselves as having limits or having a way of doing things others regard as strange or immature.

The ability to create is still one of life's greatest mysteries. It involves a tolerance for mystery and ambiguity, as well as a trust in our own abilities to understand the limitless possibilities or options which are inherent in every situation.

When there is so much positive, heartfelt energy available to us, why don't we use it more often? The answer is very simple — it's hard to think and act consistently in our own best interests when we are resentful. The old blame-and-shame game gets imbedded in our subconscious minds and we don't even know why we don't do our best.

Here is a process for getting over resentments. Even if you don't think I'm talking about you, try this process to forgive yourself and others. I know it will make a difference.

## The Forgiveness Process
* * * * * * *

Begin the forgiveness process by memorizing this Law of Blessing and saying it to yourself, preferably out loud, every time that you have the thought or feeling that you want to be forgiven for. Then, let go of it forever.

### The Law Of Blessing

*I forgive you right now*
*Wherever you are*
*Whatever you are doing*
*Whomever you are with*
*Whatever you are thinking*
*Whatever you are feeling about me or anyone else*
*I forgive you, bless you and let go of resentment.*

I have used this saying hundreds of times in my life and thousands of times with different clients. It will work because our unconscious mind is cooperative in nature and wants to respond in a positive way to wise and loving positive suggestions. All it takes to set the process in motion is a decision on your part to finally let go of the hurt you have been carrying all this time. If you have to remake the decision several times, then do it over and over. Forgiving is a proven way to get some relief.

The more baggage you are carrying, the better you will feel when you finally set it down and move on with your life. The real payoff comes when you discover how much better you feel, emotionally and physically. Those symptoms that have been signaling to you that something is wrong will slowly disappear. You may lose weight, feel less nervous, increase your tolerance for stress, look and feel younger, enjoy your present interpersonal relationships more or just be able to have more fun. It all begins with the Law of Blessing.

We forgive so we can go on with our lives. Our willingness to forgive has nothing to do with being sorry. It is a poor excuse for us to say we're unwilling to forgive someone unless they say they're sorry for what they did to us. In truth, we do ourselves a favor when we forgive because then and only then can we actually let go of a situation or person. Remember that loving and hating someone are equally powerful ways to cling to a relationship. As Zen Buddhists say, "We will be in heaven with both those we love and those we hate."

By using the power of the heart chakra to love and forgive ourselves and others, we will become free from attachments to unhealthy relationships and damaging habits of mind.

When our heart energy is no longer tied up in fear and resentment from the past, we can direct it into constructive pathways. We'll be free to develop courage, take heart, become strong within ourselves. We'll have this powerful energy available to help us create new opportunities — and follow through on making them real.

# Meditation For Love And Forgiveness

This meditation enhances our ability to love and to forgive. It helps us to let go of past failures and disgraces by channelling our energy to higher purposes in the service of others. Repeated practice helps to strengthen and bless our ability to love and forgive. It helps us serve others.

*Claim:* I will direct my energies only toward loving endeavors with others. I open my heart to love.

*Affirm:* I will behold the person whom I now consider my enemy to be, in truth, a divine friend hiding behind a veil of misunderstanding.

*Read:* "Therefore, if you bring thy gift to the altar, and there rememberest that thy brother hath ought against thee; Leave there thy gift before the altar and go thy way; first be reconciled to thy brother, and then come and offer thy gift" (Matthew 5:23-24).

*Meditation:* While sitting or lying down with your spine straight, make yourself comfortable and begin relaxing. Bathe your imagination in the green light that is centered around your heart and project this green light to all parts of your body. See this brilliant, rich light mixing with the lights from the other chakras; the red, the orange, the yellow . . . As this healing energy flows to every part of your body, let it engulf and push out any pain or discomfort. Let this brilliant light go to every dark area within and replace it with brightness and healing energy. When your breathing becomes deep and regular, repeat in cadence with your breathing, "My spirit has many gifts. The greatest of these is love." Pay attention to how the love energy moves about your body and tends to move toward others in your life.

# 7 Go With Your Inner Voice

## *The Fifth Step To Personal Power*

The fifth step to personal power entails listening to the messages of the heart, trusting them and putting them into action. As we grow up, we are taught to honor the voice of reason, to calculate, think, measure, weigh everything in a logical way and to base our lives upon such factors.

When the voice of the heart awakens, its contribution to our welfare can be profound if it comes to full expression. This takes place through the energy of the *Visuddha* chakra. Located at the base of the throat, between the mind and heart, part of the function of this powerful center is to mediate between those sometimes contradictory influences.

This center can come into its own as we move into full adulthood. If we resist the awakening heart, we may experience discomfort in the area of the throat. We may get frequent sore throats, stiff necks, chronic hoarseness or feel a lump in the throat. It's important to realize that the lump in your throat may be the voice of your heart looking for expression.

The powers of the fifth chakra are many. In the natural progression of things, this center of energy assists us and inspires us in the process of fully accepting adulthood. Located at the level of the neck behind the larynx, it influences intuition, perception, and is commonly associated with the gift of self-expression. Its color is blue. One commentator mentions that blue, the color of the cloudless sky, represents clarity. The Visuddha governs many aspects of communication with ourselves and others. It has to do with speaking and hearing, not just as purely physical abilities, but as intuitive powers of the soul.

Opening the fifth chakra allows the energy of the heart to ascend to the level of expression. We then have the potential of learning to listen with the heart and speak its truth. Often crises of adulthood have to do with listening within and following our own wisdom even when it means leaving the values of our parents and peers behind. The gift of discrimination is important at this time to help us perceive and communicate our highest truth, not as adolescent rebels but as upstanding adults.

In our meditation on this chakra we learn to turn off the chatter of our minds and understand the power of silence. As we learn to foster the ability to listen beyond words, we become attuned to that still, small voice within and the deep wisdom it communicates to us.

One noted teacher of meditation recommends concentrating on the throat chakra as a way to alleviate insomnia.

Relaxing the neck is a step toward opening the Vissudha chakra and helps bring about internal silence, quieting our own inner voice.

## Necessary Changes
* * * * * * *

Certain aspects of change are age-related and seem to be laid down in an archetypical matrix common to all people. We tend to go through major transitions approximately every 10 years, beginning at age 30. Throughout life, a natural flowering goes on, but those who are not prepared for these natural changes may think of them as crises — such as the well-known mid-life crisis. I think these transition points are only crises if we are determined to cling to how we were instead of gracefully moving on, growing as we go. The Chinese have a good perspective: Their ideogram for crisis consists of figures for both danger and opportunity.

Those of us who are terrified of natural change may get stuck in transition and never fully mature. Stuckness disempowers us. If we work too hard on pretending to be 25 when we are 45, we may create a kind of time-warp of the soul and neglect to develop our internal gifts. Our popular culture promotes the value of "staying young," but has little to offer about the benefits of maturing.

In the natural course of events, as we grow older we tend to lighten up and become more spiritual, but not all of us get there. An unmarried friend of mine in his late 30s recently joined a health club and was fascinated with how many older women were working out and looking good. But then he got worried. "They had nothing to say of any consequence. All of their attention was focused on the mirror. I began to feel as if I were in some weird sci-fi movie with beautiful robots."

I believe that staying fit and strong is a sign of good mental health, but if it becomes obsessive, it's damaging.

Neglecting inner growth in favor of externals stems from a kind of terrified self-hate and signifies rejection of self at deeper levels. On the other hand, neglecting our physical well-being while trying to master spiritual growth doesn't make sense either.

## The Fast-Forward Era
* * * * * * *

It's no secret that we are living in an age of accelerating change. Technology advances, national boundaries dissolve, economic power shifts, epidemics loom, ecological disaster threatens and who knows which megalomaniac dictator has the bomb? Add to these external changes the inevitable changes that take place inside every one of us, and our heads spin. We feel dizzy and overwhelmed with good reason. If you are over the age of 30, you've probably noticed strange things happening to your friends and colleagues. Some are making major life changes or very poor decisions, or seem to have just gone plain crazy. Psychological burnout is common and may drive them into peculiar solutions.

The average marriage now lasts only about five years. If you can count more than a few couples you know who are truly happy in their marriages, congratulations. It's sad how we enter into relationships with such high hopes for the future and before we know it, the early promise of intimacy, humor, good times and empathy has disappeared and we are frustrated by our unsuccessful attempts to make things work.

We look for explanations and excuses, read books, see therapists and may even blame our parents for our inability to have healthy relationships. Parent-bashing has been in vogue for years. When I was in graduate school, we used to chuckle that if we couldn't find out what was wrong with a client, we could always blame the parents, especially the mother. It wasn't really funny then, and still isn't an adequate diagnosis.

In my practice today the typical patient who comes in is a woman in her 30s. If she is married, she may be brought in by her husband to be "tuned up," as one would bring a car into a dealership for a 30,000 mile checkup. Whenever there is a personality or behavioral change in a woman who is simply going through a natural period of growth or change in life, there is usually a man in her life telling her something is probably wrong with her hormones. Some men seem to deliberately misunderstand a woman's desire to develop interests outside the home so they don't have to face loss of a housemaid or the challenge of their own maturing process.

As changes inevitably occur, you will benefit from learning the art of silence and listening within, especially if someone significant in your life is misinterpreting and telling you you're wrong or crazy. Developing the qualities attributed to the fifth chakra strengthens us to stave off what might be devastating damage inflicted by those who don't want us to change. As we become more centered in ourselves, disapproval (or approval) from others has less effect on us. Centering in ourselves is not the same as being self-centered. On the contrary, it gives us power to become truly selfless on behalf of other people without getting lost in the process.

## Did Someone Change The Rules?
\* \* \* \* \* \* \*

Natural shifts into different stages of life may leave you at a loss. It may seem that just when you achieve a solid sense of identity, a crisis leaves you feeling unhinged or ungrounded. As one client put it, "Just when I learned the game, they changed all the rules."

Even competent professionals suddenly seem to run out of gas, become moody and find little joy in life. Old coping strategies fail us; things that used to give pleasure or excitement no longer satisfy us. Even ownership of material goods seems lackluster.

A successful man in his late 30s came to see me because he was having panic attacks. He had no idea why he was having these attacks, but they were so bad, he would work late because he was afraid to go out into the parking lot and get into his car. He was literally frozen, overwhelmed by so much anxiety that he was unable to perform menial tasks.

## Maybe Nothing's Wrong
* * * * * * *

What goes wrong? Maybe nothing. Perhaps we just don't know enough about the natural patterns of growth and change to adapt to them gracefully.

The universal search for identity inspires books, movies and songs about the transition from a secure, optimistic life to one of psychological pain and discomfort. The theme reflects our inability to continue to identify with the kind of life we have set up for ourselves. The ego, which processes information from the external world to the inner resources of our unconscious mind and helps protect us and make good decisions, is no longer congruent with our external lives. The positive ego is ever vigilant and willing to defend and prompt us to take the best course of action. It is the driving force of our internal family.

## The Power Of Knowledge
* * * * * * *

In my workshops there are participants who say these changes don't apply to their lives and they can't relate to the material. They have no idea what I'm talking about. I always tell them to take good notes because they are sure to need them in the future. No one gets through life without going through changes, and many of them are predictable. Knowledge is power. If we know what's coming, we can be prepared to handle anything.

In Oklahoma we like to use the example of the Wise Wagon Master. When the West was still wild, wagon trains brought settlers from the East into uncharted territories. Some got through and others failed to reach their goals. The wagon masters who gained a reputation for consistently getting their wagon trains to their destinations were not known for their technical expertise but did have a very interesting characteristic in common. They communicated about the future.

Each night, they would circle the wagons around the campfire and discuss with the pioneers all the information they had gleaned from their scouts and their own observations. The weather would be harsh tomorrow, the terrain rough. Horses were dying, babies were due, the stream ahead was dry, Indians were about to attack. When people knew what to expect and prepared themselves physically, mentally, emotionally and spiritually, they had a good chance of getting through. It was not the events that would stop them, it was the *unforeseen*.

The same is true of life. Communicating change keeps us strong. If we understand both the problems headed our way from the outside and the changes scheduled on our internal calendars, we won't be caught off balance. We can become wise wagon masters of our journey through life.

## How To Recognize Signs Of Internal Shifting
★ ★ ★ ★ ★ ★ ★

When something is changing within, it feels like we are having a crisis of spirit. We may feel lost, alone in a psychological forest and experience highly charged thoughts, moods and impulses, including sexual feelings. Often we have strong intuitions, fantasies or dreams and synchronistic events take place which leave us feeling extremely psychic. It may be frightening.

Strange feelings may come on suddenly or gradually. Perhaps you feel a desperate sense of loss for no particular reason or feel defeated in some way. What was solid now seems unreal. There may be a feeling of being trapped, a growing realization of limitations and increased awareness of your limited lifespan.

We may even have a feeling of being called or led to do something we do not understand. People complain of being overwhelmed with angst: Nothing seems right anymore, they're fed up with the rat race, they lament the lack of meaning in their lives. These dreadful feelings are not permanent conditions. Rather, they are indications that something is changing — or needs to.

Two writer friends of mine in New York were always calling each other on terrible days when they felt totally bogged down. Nothing was going right, their minds were blank, they felt depressed and had no faith whatsoever that their work had any meaning or value. Before long they realized there was a pattern to these dreadful days. They invariably preceded those magical times when new thoughts would come, new ideas would surface and their writing took a great leap forward. They called them their mud days. When something was stirring the mud at the bottom of their creative ponds, they learned to put up with the discomfort and trust the process. Soon good new things would bubble to the surface.

In life as well as in art, if we can tolerate some discomfort without reaching for the tranquilizers or anti-depressants, these dreary periods of internal angst can precede major positive shifts in which a new person emerges. If we allow change to continue with awareness and without fear, we go from the mud to the clarity represented by the Visuddha chakra. We are the caterpillar turning into a beautiful butterfly. We turn over a new leaf and move into a new phase of life in which we feel whole, stable, confident and positive again.

## What Is Mid-Life?
* * * * * * *

We experience personal change in the natural course of events throughout our lives. But there are certain times when that change is enormous — at adolescence and in mid-life. I found, when writing this book, that everyone agrees that adolescence encompasses our teenage years, but most of us have our own ideas about when mid-life occurs. It has been said that mid-life has arrived when we no longer see life from a perspective of beginnings, expansions and growth, but, rather, from a perspective of ends, death, fate and limitations. Some people feel they are in mid-life at age 30, others define it as after 40 or even after 50. Perhaps they are all correct. I'm not sure everyone shares the same internal calendar. If a major loss occurs, such as an accident, illness, divorce or death of someone close, we can be thrown into this transition phase at any time in our adult lives. From now on life will never be the same — the possibility that it may eventually become better than ever seems remote. Knowing that we will face changes as we age or experience loss can help us deal intelligently with difficult times, and knowing that certain characteristics of this period are predictable helps us feel sane.

## Shift In Gender-Specific Interests
* * * * * * *

When we first begin to realize we are developing characteristics associated (at least in our minds) with the other gender, we may feel threatened. Are we real men anymore if we like to knit? Real women if we take flying lessons? If we don't know it's normal to want and need to express these new characteristics and interests, we can treat ourselves harshly. I remember becoming interested in opera and purposely taking more time to cook. Simply being at home by myself was of great comfort. These were activities I had never tried before but they were very rewarding and continue to bring me satisfaction to this day.

The creative, nurturing feminine side of my nature became more prominent and I liked it. I am certainly different now than I was when the process started.

You often see older couples who have nearly reversed roles in their relationships. He now cleans and keeps house, while she still goes to work and perhaps even takes over mowing the lawn and other jobs formerly thought to be "men's work." This is definitely a time of change. Usually a woman finds within herself the desire to express competence, to become more active in her career, finish her education or develop a more independent lifestyle.

## Meeting The Dark Side
* * * * * * *

The other part of us that comes to the surface at mid-life is our dark side, much like the Star Wars character Darth Vader. This part of us, described by Carl Jung as the shadow, gets very frustrated when we do not get our way. Sometimes minor irritations turn into full-blown rage, and we become quite vengeful. At this point our own personal evil becomes an issue, and we may throw temper tantrums. Sometimes the outbursts originating from the dark side can become far worse.

In this situation, our task is to make friends with the dark side, just as children need to make friends with the monsters in dreams because it helps them feel safer. By making friends with their monsters, they can conquer them. It is very important to understand that the fearsome part of us that seems to be evil is basically only misguided and needs to be understood, not denied. It is only trying to get our attention and believes that by surfacing in the form of anger or cruelty it is protecting us. Making friends with our shadow is a challenge we all must face.

## A Period Of Nostalgia
* * * * * * *

In times of transition, there also seems to be some kind of life review in which we become nostalgic about our childhood and may even want to visit the place where we grew up. Anger from our childhood may resurface. Any problems with our parents or nuclear family that are unresolved almost always reappear at this time to confuse us further. Because we are in a period of transition and our new self-concept is emerging, we tend to be drawn to other people who are having similar feelings. We experience an intense desire for a "soul mate" and a feeling of being called to have a relationship with someone who is like-minded.

This is also a time in life when many people change careers and feel much like a teenager again. Often there is a pervasive feeling of anger or disappointment fueled by the conviction that we are not getting the nurturing or intimacy we need. At this time of psychological distress, we are vulnerable to anything that might seduce us away from dealing with these issues. By this I mean we tend to pour ourselves into our work, to use drugs or alcohol or to do anything to release us from what we are feeling. This is also a time when we can become trapped by any of these negative behaviors or feelings. Often our spouses, or those who are close to us at the time, feel a great deal of confusion and may even blame themselves for our distress.

## An Uphill Climb
* * * * * * *

A woman I was working with gave me an excellent metaphor for talking about the stages of this transition process. She talked about always having the feeling that she was moving uphill. While she was making gradual progress toward some kind of goal or success, she recalled that it was like doggedly climbing a hill, then suddenly falling into a deep pit. It would take two or three tries to learn how to climb out and she would get muddy from every attempt to free herself.

As you read the following section about stages of transition, I would like you to imagine yourself climbing a hill, but then slipping slowly and gently down into the bottom of an oozing ditch, knowing you cannot prevent yourself from sliding into it over and over again.

The ancient Greeks knew this situation well and had a place in their pantheon for a god of quick changes. They described times of transition as a visit from Hermes, the trickster, who keeps us off guard and doesn't let us settle into too much security or comfort. Whenever we feel we have it all together, Hermes may not be far behind. Part of the wisdom of the Greeks is recognizing and making friends with Hermes. Change will come. Let's pray we'll get through it.

# The Stages Of Transition
* * * * * * *

Helen, my patient who talked about falling into the pit, also reported feeling as if she had compromised her values. Her old values no longer seem to apply to her life situation and current thinking. She recounted feeling bored, discontented with life and generally unable to accomplish anything of lasting value. She remembered that those goals she had initially set years ago of getting through graduate school, going to work in a research facility, and becoming the head of a research group, had all been realized. She believed that the real fun of it all was in the dreaming and the achieving. When she accomplished her goals, life became boring to her.

Helen's feelings signalled, in a very typical way, a transition that preceded a major life change. Similar situations often occur with very bright people and high achievers. I have come to believe that major discontent is actually the beginning of a "calling" to a new style of life. It may take two or three years to work through the series of changes necessary to complete the transition. Occasionally individuals may get stuck in one particular stage and the process will require a longer transition time.

The good news about this transition is that people can shortcut their time going through this model and, in effect, go directly to the final stage, which is one of reconstruction and spiritual awakening, if they will follow one bit of simple advice: Go immediately within yourself.

The model for this transition looks like a cross-section of a ditch with a great big self in the middle. This self can be seen as the core of psychological being, the soul, the spiritual essence and the innermost part of any person. Each of us goes through these stages to some extent — to a large extent, if we ignore our inner spiritual calling, and to a small extent, if we delve into ourselves and confront our own sense of purpose and allow the "new" self to emerge.

In our late teens or early 20s, we often set goals for ourselves which we steadily work toward until they are achieved. Sometimes we find we are tracking along on automatic pilot, with little self-awareness or sense of direction. There are two common situations that can pull us up short and cause major shifts in our attitudes and outlook. The first one is a crisis that nearly overwhelms us. This can be the death of a loved one, loss of a job or an injury that drastically affects our lives from now on. Because of this crisis, life is now different for us than ever before. The second circumstance is achievement of our goals and the unexpected feelings of hopelessness and sadness resulting from that completion.

Alexander the Great was said to have sat down and wept when he had no more countries to conquer. When

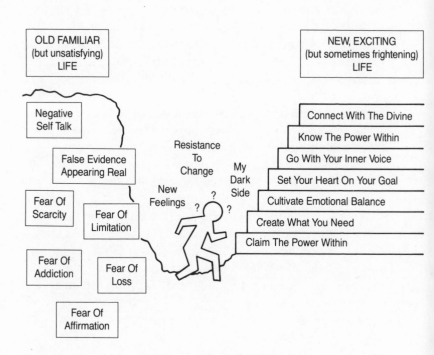

**Figure 7.1. Into The "Pits"**

we encounter such hopelessness and discouragement, we generally think back to the times when we were happy, and recall what once gave us a sense of purpose and mission. When this sense is missing, we can slip into the pits in predictable stages. The five fears discussed in Chapter 2 take over, and we can feel trapped.

## Common Transitional Stages
\* \* \* \* \* \* \*

For some reason, there is a cultural prejudice against speaking about the transitional changes of our lives, as if one should be embarrassed for showing signs of "weakness." Locking into shame about going through the transitions of adulthood is a perfect psychological killer from which we may not recover. The danger comes when people feel bewildered or ashamed, go underground and suffer in silence. Such people may never get through it or over it, and their lives may deteriorate steadily.

When clients suffering from mid-life malaise finally come into the office, they breathe a deep sigh of relief when they learn that what they are going through is typical of most people. "Why didn't somebody tell me?" they commonly exclaim. "If I had known, life would have been much easier for everyone concerned."

The most common transitional stages are the overly conventional stage, the rebel stage, the falling apart stage, the reconstruction stage, the sacrifice-and-change stage and the stage of reintegrating spiritual resources.

### 1. The Overly Conventional Stage

At first we might turn back and try to recapture whatever gave us pleasure and purpose in the past. For men, this is often a time when they tend to get reinvolved in some kind of social club or community endeavor, buy a new three-piece suit and attempt to get back to the characteristics to which they attribute their success. Women may go through a *House Beautiful* stage and lavish attention on home improvement. They may attempt to get reinvolved with their children who are now older and may not relish the mother's renewed interest. Both men and women may become rigid and try to keep tight control over everything to maintain the status quo. After these attempts to yield the hoped-for return to happiness fail, the second stage is ushered in.

## 2. The Rebel Stage

The second stage is one of rebellion and is generally referred to as the "middle-aged crazies." This is a time when people feel irritable and angry full-time. They may feel rebellious toward authority and want to dump the whole package of their lives. Perhaps you know someone who, apparently for no reason, stops having anything to do with you. This is because you are a part of the "package" that the person is attempting to unload. During this time people seem to compromise their values, purchase things they associate with their youth (such as sporty cars they cannot afford) and become vulnerable to the influences of anything that they believe will make them feel better or younger. When I went through this stage, the only thing I could imagine would bring me any happiness was a vintage 1950 Packard sedan. Rebellion toward authority gives people problems on the job, as well as difficulty meeting the responsibilities they have eagerly accepted in the past.

Sometimes a new look seems to be in order. People get a new hairstyle, a new wardrobe and start associating with an entirely different group of people, leaving behind those they have been with before. Often a person is said to be making a fool of himself or herself and people talk about how much the individual has changed.

Both men and women try to go back to what they know. Men who achieved much in life may revert to hanging out at a corner saloon with drinking buddies who are not in their league at all, but remind them of the good old days when they first started out. Women commonly emulate their mothers whether or not they are suitable models.

## 3. The Falling Apart Stage

The third stage is one of falling apart when the "this-is-not-working" attitude evolves. Depression and pessimism set in. In this stage the individual often becomes more accident prone. When I recognize this tendency in my clients, I plead with them to put on their seat belts, look both ways before pulling into an intersection and take whatever extra measures they can to insure their own personal safety. It is at times like this when people lapse into secret love affairs, have business failures, become ill and very often change jobs. The individual changes his or her whole life when the old life falls apart, and a new one has not yet been put together. It is very painful to see a loved one go through this kind of ordeal, which sometimes culminates in emotional, financial and physical bankruptcy.

## 4. The Reconstruction Stage

The fourth stage of life reconstruction begins with the admission that life isn't working and the intention of putting it back together. The problem is, some people cannot surrender to making that admission. In 12-Step groups dedicated to putting lives back together, the first step is always to admit life is unmanageable. (Most people are unaware that the 12-Step process is a spiritual life plan that predates Alcoholics Anonymous by centuries.) In the Baptist church as well as others, it is said you must surrender your will to God when something traumatic happens.

For those who cannot surrender their ego in some way, life reconstruction may never happen. If they don't begin the real nuts and bolts work of building their lives, they become vulnerable and may fall prey to crazy get-rich-quick schemes, con men and various forms of addiction.

## 5. The Sacrifice-And-Change Stage

This stage indicates the need to take inventory and, perhaps, incorporate major changes into our lifestyle. Very often people begin a new career and relocate to new geographical areas or neighborhoods. Their inward change is manifesting in external forms and they may adopt a more attractive look in the way that they dress. Sometimes they even become serious about getting into shape physically. This is also a time when the creative juices begin to flow and the individual begins to do things such as write, learn to play a musical instrument, paint, redecorate their living quarters or do anything that signals a change.

## 6. The Reintegration-Of-Spiritual-Resources Stage

The true characteristic of this stage is turning inward to delve into our spiritual resources. This stage is characterized by an intensified spiritual life, a deepening of interpersonal relationships and a new self-awareness. There is less projection and blaming and more self-confident acceptance of who we are and what we want in life. Usually the soul moves into high gear, generating opportunities and options.

The spiritual part of us can now identify with the new self, and the ego part of us is now willing to work at helping us set new goals, accomplish new things and find new ways of serving. A new consciousness of spirituality develops, yet at the same time, life seems to become more real.

## 7. Other Aspects Of The Transition Model

After the reintegration stage, a new spiritual person evolves. Life can take on an entirely new meaning at this point, yet we may still be tempted to sell ourselves short and not go the full distance with this transition. Sometimes, to grasp at security, people are tempted either to get into a new relationship or get out of an old one. At this stage, some therapists might persuade a person to retreat, regress or go back to the point where they were a couple of years earlier. They might even bring a lot of heavy moral judgment to bear upon the patient to stop them from changing.

I know of one therapist who had a reputation for being a "wife killer." He worked with women whose husbands did not like the changes they were going through and persuaded them to stay in denial stage, negating their urge to grow. All this was for the convenience of, or at the request of, the husbands who did not want their wives to change or become confident. I question his ethics.

One of the funniest things I hear from spouses is, "I don't know what's the matter with Harry. He just isn't the person I married!" This statement while hilarious is also rather tragic. The idea that we are supposed to remain exactly as we were, changing little as we go through life, is absolutely ludicrous. Yet people tend to think that if their partner does change, something drastic has happened. They feel uncomfortable unless the person immediately reverts to their old familiar ways.

## The Family's Reaction To Change
* * * * * * *

There are three things that will almost always happen to the person who is on the road to transition. First, their friends, colleagues or families will say they are wrong. The second is that these same people will ask, or demand, that the person change back to the way they were. If that doesn't work they will up the ante and say, "Change back or I'll . . ." They make threats and imply that if they continue on this growth or adventure path, they are going to be rejected by those who should be most supportive. What inevitably happens to the ones who are compromised is that they develop an additional set of symptoms.

A woman in a major transition thought she could function in a healthy way in her marriage, but her husband did not like her getting a job and becoming "too religious." He repeatedly told her she was wrong, and eventually put pressure on her to terminate therapy or to see another therapist who was more sympathetic to his desires for her. He refused to come into sessions with her because he did not want to have to deal with her changes.

She and I discussed this problem at length many times. She finally decided that it was not worth fighting him. She would give up her career, go back to staying at home with him, stop writing poetry and take the heavy dose of anti-depressants the other professional had recommended for her. She stopped coming for our sessions and began taking the medication.

I had not talked to this woman for approximately two years when I happened to meet her daughter unexpectedly. The daughter told me that her mother had indeed gone back to live the life her father had demanded. She also told me that her mother had been diagnosed with cancer and was not expected to live for more than a few months. If communication from our inner voice requires us to change, ignoring its directives can sometimes be fatal — as it was in this case.

## Grow Or Shrink
* * * * * * *

I can recite incident after incident like this from 20 years of experience. If we do not allow ourselves to follow through on change, the results can be disastrous, if not potentially fatal. It is very interesting to me how our expectations determine the patterns of our lives, when, in reality, we can easily make choices. We can develop, grow, create and become more spiritually inspired or we can become accepting of a lesser fate and wither on the vine. It almost seems that we are driven to make intelligent choices. Hermes, trickster that he is, can lead us into paths of bliss and ecstasy or he can kill us, depending on what we choose.

If we allow the natural process of change to occur and learn to access the subtle powers of the fifth chakra, we find new spaces of silence within. We bring forth new voices and listen to our new selves with love. We can listen better to each other and our relationships may improve.

## A Different Self
* * * * * * *

The series of transitions we have been through finally comes full circle and stability once again returns. We sense the return of normalcy, but it's a different kind of normal. Our spiritual life has deepened, and we have more self-confidence. We have learned to trust the inner voice of our hearts. Our spirit has now been put into service in our quest for growth, and enlightenment is the goal of our quest rather than material gain.

The real paradox of our quest for spirit and meaning is that, when we reach this spiritual plateau, we may become more successful financially and in every other way than we have ever been before, and feel we have really found our place in the world. Generally people are happier with their lives and have a stronger sense of belonging than ever before.

## Who Guides The Process Of Change?
* * * * * * *

The best guides are those who have been through this "trial by fire" themselves and who are able to guide other people through. After surviving the experience themselves, they have gained immeasurable insight.

Transition is a time when one has to be very forgiving both of self and others who are going through the process. Families and those close to people making a major change should be aware that they should have two months to be totally crazy without any condemnation from those who love them. It is very important to be forgiving.

Look for a counselor who is a combination therapist and spiritual guide and who is comfortable with the spiritual sytem that holds promise for you. Find someone who has compassion, creativity and heart. A dash of humor also wouldn't hurt. I tell clients to learn to laugh at themselves and be more objective about what is happening to them. They need to be prepared for the strong surges of feeling that occasionally overwhelm. I also try to help them risk and live while feeling vulnerable, knowing that things will get better. At the same time, I must advise them to protect themselves in their vulnerability.

Getting involved in new activities with new friends helps, but it is not advisable to succumb to the temptation to trade security for chaos. I encourage clients to deepen their long-term relationship and not trade the temporary intimacy of an affair for the opportunity to strengthen a marriage. While each individual must set personal priorities, the two as a couple must also have mutual goals to strive for. Each needs to realize that change is inevitable and basically it will be beneficial to both in the long run.

Change is interfered with when people turn to drugs, including psychotropics prescribed by well-meaning physicians. Instant relief leaves them unmotivated to struggle with the changes that are going on within them. They become blocked. The chakra energy cannot flow. The Holy Spirit cannot reach them.

## How To Keep From Falling Apart
* * * * * * *

How do we stop ourselves from going through the whole cycle? Must we fall apart and lose everything before we can move to the stage of reintegration and spiritual renewal? The answer is an emphatic "No!" Three things are needed to help any person through these transition stages:

1. Find someone to share your thoughts and feelings with. One way to do this is psychotherapy.
2. Keep busy with projects that will help you expand your areas of personal interest.
3. Accept and forgive yourself and others.

Without these key elements, you will certainly get stuck in transition and may become physically or mentally ill.

The way to keep from falling into the pits is to develop a spiritual bridge. Attending religious services, exploring religious symbolism, meditating, praying and seeking out spiritual literature, tapes and movies can ease the transition process. I stress developing spiritual interests to clients since I know they will descend to rebellion and disintegration if they fail to explore the spiritual. In the Appendix there is a list of books, tapes and movies I have used with good results to help guide patients gently through spiritual confusion.

## What Has Really Changed?
* * * * * * *

After all the time, worry, fear and trauma of shifting into our mature selves, we may look back and wonder what happened. When all is said and done we have gone through a difficult process to achieve only a small change: Our doors of perception are opened. We may look in the mirror and see ourselves as not very different but once we cross the threshold into wholeness (and holiness), we can't go back. We have unleashed the power within. Using the example of a TV dial, we have moved only one click away, but found a whole new world.

Necessary changes in life can only come about when we learn to listen within, trust ourselves and act on our

inner whisperings. We are more fully whole and well in
every sense of the word.

## Self-Analysis
* * * * * * *

Ask yourself the following questions frequently to stay
on the right path:

1. Are you listening to your inner voice? Honoring your
   personal truth?
2. What is happening to friends, their lives, marriages
   and careers? Do many of their concerns mirror much
   of your own life?
3. Are your goals clear? Are you running out of goals?
   Who do you talk with about goals?
4. How are you handling crises in your life? Are there
   any future crises coming up (children leaving, a parent dying, career change, financial change)?
5. How is your spiritual life? Is it alive and real? Are
   you nurturing your spiritual needs?
6. What have you done or are you doing to nurture
   your spirit?
7. What have you done today or this week to nurture
   your spirit through meditation, prayer and study?

REMEMBER: Being able to examine your life in terms
of these fundamental questions is a big part of staying
fine-tuned and healthy.

# Meditation For Going With The Voice Within

This meditation helps us focus energy on communicating to ourselves and to others. The energy from the fifth chakra is one of discovery and communication. Repeated practice helps us to focus our attention on what it is that we wish to express in any situation.

*Claim:* I will learn to communicate better with others by first learning to listen more clearly within myself.

*Affirm:* Beginning with the early dawn each day, I will radiate joy to everyone I meet. I will be mental sunshine for all who cross my path. I will burn candles of smiles and darkness will take flight.

*Read:* "Ask and it shall be given to you. Seek and ye shall find. Knock and it shall be opened unto you" (Matthew 7:7).

*Meditation:* Sit up straight in a comfortable chair or lie down with your spine straight. Close your eyes and take a few deep breaths. Pay attention to your neck and throat. Bring relaxation to this area. Visualize a cool and refreshing blue light emanating from your throat chakra. See this light spiraling around to other areas of your body and mixing with every one of the lower chakra lights. See this light reaching to every part of your conscious and

unconscious mind, clearing networks of communication patterns between and among all of your
different parts. Let this blue light rise into your
head and out the top, spilling out and flowing down
over you.

When your breathing becomes deep and regular,
repeat for three minutes to the rhythm of your
breath, "I am willing to honor my true inner voice
with love and respect." As you do this, pay attention to any part of you that seems to desire to
communicate and listen carefully to any aspect of
your being that seems to want your attention or
support.

# CHAPTER

# 8 Know The Power Within

## The Sixth Step To Personal Power

Sagacity is not a word we use often in Western culture, but in the Oriental world and among indigenous peoples, those who have lived consciously are looked up to as sages. Wisdom is revered.

If we accept the lessons of the first five steps to personal power, we come to the highest power of the human mind represented by the sixth chakra. In Sanskrit the name of this chakra is *Ajna*, meaning *to know, perceive and command*. It is located at a point between the eyebrows, and its color is deep indigo blue.

With development of this center, we reach the highest power of the human mind. Wisdom and understanding are refined and we achieve the ability to see beyond circumstances. Even if we do nothing to develop this center, it becomes stronger as we age and accumulate knowledge from personal experience, but we can learn to develop wisdom if we practice one-pointed mind. Intense powers of concentration are associated with genius, but can be developed by anyone with average intelligence who has the will to meditate and focus on this center.

When attainment of intense mental powers is combined with love and intuition, the hopes and dreams of all mankind can be served. If we aspire to wisdom to create abundance on earth, we can bridge the material and spiritual worlds. The energies of the sixth chakra represent the highest development of human beings. Beyond this level of attainment, everything depends on the Divine.

One of the most important factors in creating personal power and opportunities for a better life is to find what brings you bliss. You may have heard the phrase "follow your bliss," usually attributed to mythologist Joseph Campbell, but what does it really mean and why is it so important?

In India disciples describe the nature of the Supreme Reality as *Satchitananda*. Its meaning is expressed in its three syllables: *Sat* is *Being*, that which exists in all times, in all places and in all things; *Chit* is *Consciousness*, that which illumines all things; and *Ananda* is supreme *Bliss*, that which gives full delight. Holy teachers, or gurus, are given names that end in "ananda," signifying attainment of the bliss state of consciousness. For example, the name *Amritananda* is a combination of *amrit*, which means sweetness or inner nectar, and *ananda*. A woman called Mata Amritananda is a guru who radiates the holiness of love and sweetness. Her name represents what she *is*. Her disciples are imbued with her powerful energy without doing anything to get it, an excellent example of the power generated by someone following her bliss.

# The Nature Of Bliss

* * * * * * *

What is your bliss? Think for a minute about what really turns you on, exhilarates and helps you experience an extraordinary feeling that may approach the Divine. Your bliss may reveal itself in quiet times when you are alone.

I once worked with an executive who appeared to be very successful, but his success was marred by unhappiness with his work. He had created one of the best-known and respected businesses in the Midwest. Yet in the midst of his financial success, he complained of being bored, having no challenges other than those provided by the humdrum existence of his daily work. He said that he was beginning to feel like a phony because he could advise everyone else how to handle their circumstances and problems, but when it came down to his own problems, he really did not know what would make him happy. I told him that he *did* know what he wanted to do, but he had not given himself permission to do it.

I was right. He said he did have a dream and already had a plan to accomplish it. Still, he was holding himself back emotionally. He believed he would be unable to sell his present business and his house. If he could be assured of selling these two enormous investments, he would, in his own words, "leave tomorrow."

I advised him to go ahead and move, and told him he would be amazed that his house would sell as soon as he had made a 100 percent commitment. Move, and obstacles would disappear. Six months later he came back. It was the middle of the summer and the pressure was on. He had school-age children who needed to be in place by the time school began in the fall.

In our second session he again spoke of how badly he wanted to move and his desire to undertake this venture in another state. In spite of all this, he still had been unable to get up the nerve to pursue his dream until his business and house were sold. He had several lookers, he confessed, but none of them seemed genuinely interested. I reminded him once again of the effect of a 100 percent commitment, and gently tried to convince him that things would, indeed, fall into place for him. He was no exception to this universal truth.

I told him I would raise the fee for my counseling service if he would not listen to my advice. He assured me he would take my advice and he promised to call if he needed to talk further. In a week he called to say he had taken a leap of faith and purchased a home in the other state. Two days later he called again, this time with the news that the first person who had looked at his business bought it and also purchased his home. He was moving within the month.

This story is not unusual in any sense of the word. In my experience it repeats time after time. Once you make a real commitment and sign your name on the dotted line, things will begin falling into place. The only requirement is that you do what you love, follow your bliss.

It is tempting to talk about making one's own reality based on faith. But I believe that this universal principle is based on experience, rather than faith. If you will simply act upon your own experience, things will follow a natural progression.

## Stop Working Now
\* \* \* \* \* \* \*

Many people have turned hobbies they love into new careers. An old adage about seeking a vocation says you should simply find out what you really like to do (your bliss), then determine how to make a living doing it. That way you will never have to work another day in your life!

Many writers have dealt with the problems of not following one's bliss. Nietzsche, a famous German philosopher, spoke of three necessary transformations of the spirit. In our first youthful state, we are camels. We are obedient and go into the desert as we have been taught. In the second state, we are transformed into lions whose purpose is to kill the dragon called "thou shalt." The more obedient the camel, the stronger the lion will be. When the lion kills the dragon, the lion then transforms into a child and life truly begins.

The more obedient children are at first, the more likely they are to gain strength and wisdom, to be good stewards of their power, and to use it wisely when they become lions. The lion, for all of its strength, must eventually throw off society's demands and become as a child again, doing what it wants to do, being loved and nurtured for who it is. Change is predicated on first being an obedient camel, then becoming a powerful lion.

## Spiritual Growth Stages
* * * * * * *

The Sanskrit model *Satchitananda* demonstrates stages of spiritual growth. It is the brink, the jumping-off place to the ocean of transcendence. At first, *Sat* represents the bliss of just being and appreciating the opportunity to be alive, enjoying everyday living.

*Chit* is the bliss of being fully conscious or aware, fully congruent on the inside and outside, attuned to yourself and others. Awareness of others and your reaction to them is in balance. In the healing arts, it is very important for healers to be fully aware of their own feelings, thoughts and pains.

*Ananda* is bliss, rapture, transcendence, ecstasy. Though these states may only be attained fully by realized masters who focus their entire energies on achieving such spiritual highs, we can experience moments of bliss with chanting, dancing, laying on of hands (or having them laid on) or taking the Eucharist (Holy Communion).

Moments of bliss transcend this world and show us something of the Divine.

## Stay In The Now, Leave Pain Behind
* * * * * * *

We commonly live in three dimensions: the past, the present and the future. When we are in pain, "dark" grief and feelings of depression come as we mentally live in the past, think about losses, grief and wounds we have sustained. Then there are "bright" bad feelings, such as fear and panic. These are almost always linked to living in the future. Both types of pain can be alleviated by concentrating and living entirely in the present.

As psychologists like to say, if you have one foot in the past and the other in the future, then it is very likely that you will end up in the present — on your rear.

I am absolutely convinced that following your bliss has as much to do with living in the present as it does with honoring your intuition and joy. When you follow your bliss, you would swear you are helped by hidden hands. People who share your interests pop up. Your services are in demand.

## Follow The Trail To Bliss
* * * * * * *

If following bliss is so easy, why aren't we all doing it? Why do some of us never seem to accomplish exactly what we really want? In the 1940s researchers experimented to determine how people and animals resolve conflicts. They observed how all kinds of organisms approached something they wanted badly. They discovered that when a person or animal is on the brink of getting what they long for, two distinct sets of feelings begin to evolve. The first is positive feelings that seem to increase as the subject gets closer and closer to the goal. Just before the goal is reached, however, an equally strong set of negative feelings evolve and increase in strength. Eventually, these two lines intersect. Beyond that point, more negative feelings are experienced than positive. The point at which the positive and negative feelings are equal is called the point of indecision. Usually if we are able to push back resistance and move ahead to the goal, negative feelings will quickly disappear and positive feelings will increase.

Once we realize that having negative feelings does not mean we have made a bad choice, most of us can proceed through the negative feelings to the positive. Things get better after we get through our initial fright or other negative feelings. Unless we understand how our feelings will change as goals are attained, most of us will push the goal further into the future. That way, we go back to a time where we only have positive feelings and no negative feelings about it at all. We keep imagining how wonderful it will be as long as it is actually not imminent.

It is very important to go right on through the negativity that always accompanies pursuit of our goals.

## Understanding Your Dreams
* * * * * * *

For eons, humankind has believed that God directly interprets things for us and guides us through our dreams. Biblical writings indicate that people have always been interested in their own dreams and the meaning they have found in them. One of the most fascinating things we can do to gain better understanding of our bliss — and what keeps us from it — is to analyze our dreams. I am frequently asked to interpret the dreams of people who assume that their dream has only one meaning, that its meaning is very obscure and that it requires an expert to interpret. These are absolutely false notions. Anyone can learn to analyze their own dreams. To get started, record your dreams in a journal. In addition to writing your dreams in a journal, write down your reflections and thoughts about them.

There are many different kinds of dreams. Some are merely unconscious, random pieces of information, similar to static on a radio. Probably they mean very little. Even the unconscious mind needs to be given free expression once in a while. Some of my colleagues would disagree. They believe that any dream content is worth exploring. Working with any kind of dream will be an adventure, but static-like, data-processing dreams have less to offer.

If you are interested in exploring dreams, I recommend working with a tape recorder or pencil and paper next to the bed. If you ask yourself to wake up and remember your dream, you probably will. I use my dream time as a way of solving problems. I often go to sleep with a problem for my unconscious mind to work on so that I can have an answer by the next morning. Many years ago I taught statistics and research design. When I would get stumped on a problem, I would literally sleep on it and frequently come up with a workable solution in my dream.

The most important dreams tend to be those which recur. It seems the deep consciousness is willing to repeat it until you understand its message. The language of dreams is foreign to most of us because we are not accustomed to talking to ourselves using symbols or metaphors. Those of us who have adopted a new nationality sometimes get very clear messages in our native tongue.

We may forget our dreams, but all of us have them. It's worthwhile to be curious about dreams and to consider them metaphors for our inner truth. When we use a metaphor to describe a personal problem, our emotional link to the problem is removed and we can look at the situation and understand our options better. We can create new opportunities with the messages our dreams toss up on the shores of our conscious minds.

Here is an excellent system for interpreting dreams. Use the following chart to record your dreams.

## Chart 1. Dream Chart

| Dream Elements | Phrases & Qualities | Feelings | Thoughts |
|---|---|---|---|
| List elements of your dream<br><br>#1 | "I dreamed...."<br>"I am...."<br>"I see...." | "I feel...."<br>(A feeling can be described in no more than 2 words, list several feelings occurring at once) | "I think...."<br>(A thought is a sentence or description that is generated as a concept of the situation as a whole) |
| #2 | | | |
| #3 | | | |
| #4 | | | |
| #5 | | | |
| #6 | | | |
| What do these items individually represent to you? | Use a first person description as if you *are* acting the dream element or person. Retell the story from this perspective. | Note the sequence of feeling states. Are they familiar? What do they mean to you? | What do you think it means? Does it correspond to something going on in your life? |

Gestalt theory, which I find useful, suggests that everything in your dreams is you. Therefore, you are the most
appropriate person to interpret the message. Any interpretation you make of a dream's symbolism and meaning
is acceptable and correct. Here is a dream told to me by a
young man who had recently been through a divorce. He
had come to me because he was having difficulty getting
involved with people socially and had become more with-
drawn since the time of his divorce. He was very hurt
because he blamed himself for his wife's alcoholism. He
felt he was partially responsible because he never paid
any attention to her, yet insisted that she not do anything
for herself. He had always denied he had been much of an
influence in her life.

The young man dreamed that he was on a train full of
people. As time went on, more and more people got off
the train, and the terrain became increasingly desolate.
The train moved up and down hills, and finally ran out of
track in the middle of nowhere. When it came to a stop in
a desert, the young man found that the train had neither
an engineer nor a conductor. He was totally and undeni-
ably alone.

When he looked at this dream, he was convinced that it
depicted how he was cutting people out of his life, as,
indeed, he had been for some time by pouring himself
into his research. That might have been the end of the
interpretation, but I felt we should continue by filling out
the chart.

When you use this chart, first record or write your
dream in first person in the present tense. Then go to the
second column and tell how you felt after the dream.

It is important to get to the feeling level and not get
stuck in thoughts. A feeling can be described in less than
two words. A thought needs a sentence or a much longer
description.

Now look at the sequence of feelings. Inevitably when
they use this chart, people discover sequences of feelings

## Chart 2. Dream Chart Completed

| Dream Elements | Phrases & Qualities | Feelings | Thoughts |
|---|---|---|---|
| #1 Self | I dreamed about a train. I am a passenger. I see people, track, mountains, and desert. | - Not in control<br>- Observing<br>- Alone, hurt | - Confused<br>- Along for the ride<br>- Unfamiliar area |
| #2 Train | No engineer, No conductor | Helpless | What is going to happen? |
| #3 People | Full of people that keep getting off | Confused, hurt | People don't like me |
| #4 Mountains | Are tall and insurmountable | Overwhelmed | A lot of trouble to scale them |
| #5 Desert | Middle of nowhere | Isolated, alone | No one can help me |
| #6 Track | Ran out of track | Alone | Am I cutting people out of my life? |
| What do these items individually represent to you? | Use a first person description as if you *are* acting the dream element or person. Retell the story from this perspective. | Note the sequence of feeling states. Are they familiar? What do they mean to you? | What do you think it means? Does it correspond to something going on in your life? |

that seem to cluster together and keep repeating. In fact, one of the first things I ask the dreamer to tell me about during our initial interview is what seems to be happening over and over in his or her life. If certain events happen over and over in your life, they are reflected at the level of repeated sequences of feelings in your dreams. You can get valuable clues about how you are disempowering yourself at a subconscious level.

The man who dreamed of the train ride revealed many things about himself that were much more important and relevant than the simple analysis that he initially gave about his dream. In fact, this man's dream revealed certain aspects of his personality dynamics which he never thought about before: the specific way that people seemed to leave him, the method by which he seemed to drive them away, the sequence of his bad feelings and how this sequence of feelings almost always left him feeling helpless. This chain of events results in his losing control and resigning himself to the idea that these things always happen to him.

When we uncovered these hidden attitudes, we were able to find ways to break into this negative pattern that kept him alone. You can apply the power of your conscious mind to the problems of the unconscious mind and bring them into harmony. When you take this step toward achieving single-mindedness, you release energy and increase your power.

## Are You Thinking Or Feeling?
* * * * * * *

How do we misuse the extraordinary power of our mind? By tying it up with negative emotions that occlude our intelligence. You can get out of that rut by determining whether they are "thinking" or "feeling" problems. The *Diagnostic and Statistical Manual of Mental Disorders (DSM-III-R)* is broken down into these dimensions. There is much overlapping between thinking and feeling. We can conceptualize a continuum with "thinking" on one side and "feeling" on the other. Most of the time we tend to weave these two threads of mental process into a series of thoughts or feelings, or a combination of thought and feeling to form an idea.

It is always helpful to ask ourselves two questions about any problem: The first question is, "What do I *think* about it?" and the other question is "How do I *feel* about it?" It is important to know if we are in a thinking mode or in a feeling mode, because the two are as different as are their outcomes. Problems are brought about by not knowing the difference. Many people who have been victims of physical or sexual abuse have compound problems. When children have been abused, they almost always erect a defense structure which involves the use of one mode (either thinking or feeling) to the exclusion of the other. For most of us, decision-making involves unconsciously taking a mental inventory of how we think and feel about the situation.

Survivors of abuse have a difficult time creating opportunities for themselves because their choice is limited to either thinking or feeling. Depending on the intensity of the abuse, they have a difficult time bringing these two together. Abuse does not make sense. Those who have been abused learn to cope with the non-sense of abuse by separating thinking and feeling from each other. They cannot put together an acceptable rationale for being abused, except to conclude that they are very bad and *deserve* to be abused. Trying to believe lies takes its toll and leads to the fracturing of an individual's personality. Sometimes even multiple personality problems can evolve. The thinking and feeling aspects of abuse cannot be reconciled in a child's mind. Thus, the child teaches himself to either think or feel, but never to integrate the two. The legacy of abuse is an impaired ability to solve problems.

You enter the road to recovery when you ask yourself how you think and feel regarding any situation.

# The Power Of Gradual Change

\* \* \* \* \* \* \*

When we speak of creating opportunities, remember to bring about a little bit of change at a time and then nurture it to keep it growing. Gradual change is more likely to last. Consider rowing a boat across a lake. You can intentionally change the direction of the boat several degrees, without immediately noticing any difference in where you are heading. As you get closer to shore, however, you realize that you will land far from the destination you chose before making that seemingly small mid-course adjustment. Most of us operate on automatic pilot in our lives. We make a correction and try to maintain the adjustment, but the automatic pilot kicks in and before we know it, we're drifting back to doing things exactly the way we did them before.

Your automatic pilot can be shut off if you faithfully make those small course adjustments and then keep them alive.

We are creatures of habit. We say that we want to change, but do not actually relish the idea. Change causes a potential disruption in our lives. I have even seen people cry when they leave a battle zone, get out of prison or abandon a very destructive and degrading relationship. A part of us really *wants* to hang on to the old — no matter how bad it has been. We come a long way in our development when we can actually embrace change as a positive option in our lives.

Often those who have worked hard all their lives or who consider themselves to be self-made have the hardest time giving up anything or taking any kind of risk. They feel that if they let up or do anything for themselves, then they are apt to lose everything that they have worked so hard to accomplish. These people almost always have rigid defense mechanisms which send up warning flags to let them know that what they are about to do may get them into trouble. When someone has an extremely strong exterior, chances are it blankets a very frightened individual within.

There is a very subtle way we talk ourselves out of our bliss without even gaining any real knowledge of it. Because we are often too quick to stop ourselves from getting into potentially dangerous circumstances, we miss out on many good things in life. We are simply too afraid to take the risk involved. Even though we say we want to change, another channel is playing inside our heads saying no. Negative self-talk can keep you stuck in the status quo.

Be sure you have your own permission to grow. If you speak to yourself in negative terms, chances are you are canceling many of the good things you are trying to do for yourself. Remember to speak to yourself only in positive terms. The next time you ask yourself *not* to do something, you are setting up a "conscious versus unconscious" conflict within your mind. Try to avoid negative action words such as *don't, won't, shouldn't, couldn't, haven't,* and *weren't* when you talk to yourself. You must be careful about what you are actually requesting from your unconscious mind.

## Back To Square One
* * * * * * *

In our pursuit of bliss, we may get confused. What are we doing? Where are we going? In these instances, I would encourage you to go back to square one. Ask yourself the following questions and consider your responses:

- "What is it that I am trying to accomplish here?"
- "What is it that I want?"
- "How can I begin to cope with this situation?"

If I personally get muddled in any way during a therapy session, I always go back to square one, asking the client what we are working on now and what our goal, or desired outcome is for this situation. Often I find that one of us has changed our focus or gone off the track. Anytime I feel that I am not tracking or have lost empathy, I check it out. I ask myself the same questions each time:

- "What am I doing?"
- "What are the goals?"
- "Am I really listening?"

Always remember to understand that when we discover our bliss, we are more in tune with obeying universal law than at any other time, and are likely to get help from unseen hands. While bliss needs to be in the service of others, it also needs to arise from our own hearts. Without these two qualities, our quest will not come to fruition.

In most of the major religions and philosophies of the world, those who eventually achieve their goals have done two very important things on an ongoing and consistent basis. First they have compiled a list of their goals and kept this list near them at all times. They also keep an object nearby which is a powerful symbol of the goal. They may even have duplicates of it at home and at work, so they are constantly reminded of what they hope to achieve. Second, achievers work on a daily basis to move closer to the realization of that goal. It is very important that *something*, no matter how minor, be done *daily* toward attaining your goal. If it is not worked toward daily, the goal loses its importance. Then your yearning for the goal gradually subsides. In essence, the original goal becomes less desirable and may be abandoned.

## Our Goals Need Updating
* * * * * * *

If we address our goals consistently, they eventually demand action of some kind, either to accelerate, decelerate or abandon them. Few of us really work at our goals enough for them to become active and vibrant parts of our living. A goal becomes reality only if you *think* about it, frequently *remind* yourself of it and *do* something every day to achieve it. It is just that simple.

In Lewis Carroll's *Alice in Wonderland*, the Cheshire Cat announced, "If you don't care where you are going, then it doesn't matter which way you walk. You'll get somewhere if you only walk long enough." Many people lack the belief that their goals can ever be achieved and prefer to live by fate. If you do not set goals and work toward them daily, you will undoubtedly wind up "somewhere." But is it where you want to be?

Social scientists agree that we all have a great capacity for creativity and learning, yet few of us are actually living up to our own potential for achieving whatever it is that we really want. We lack a faith in ourselves and in our own potential. To see whether you are living up to your potential, sit down every January and write out at least five goals to be accomplished within five years. Do this in a spirit of sincerity and commitment. Working toward the goal is always easier when the goal itself involves something that we believe in that is larger than ourselves. Our goals should stretch our abilities beyond our personal limitations.

## Setting Goals As We Mature
\* \* \* \* \* \* \*

We never lose our need for goal-setting. At any age we can make the most of what we have, to live out our potential. The secret to coping successfully with aging and its changes is to realize that your body is only an instrument, a source of energy and spirituality. By keeping this attitude in mind, we can grow old gracefully and accept physical changes with little regret. When we can let go of our bodies psychologically, the real issues of life can be emphasized. People who are dying cut through red tape quickly and move immediately to what is important to them. Whenever we experience limits such as those imposed upon us by a deteriorating body, we rapidly make adjustments to bring into focus those things which are truly important and have lasting value to us.

## The Joy Of The Universal Connection
* * * * * * *

In *Super Joy*, Paul Pearsall describes working with a Holocaust victim whose biggest concern, while imprisoned, was not whether she had enough to eat, but whether she would lose her ability to experience real joy. The woman tells of taking her very meager food rations one day and giving them to the guard dog to eat. Everyone around her thought that she had gone completely insane, but she wanted to see if she could still enjoy watching a dog (similar to a once beloved pet) eating and somehow still feel connected to her nurturing side. Her behavior might have seemed very strange, but she realized if she could feel the wholeness she felt at a happy time in her life, she was not spiritually dead.

As we grow, we come to understand that it is joy for joy's sake that we seek. Then we are better able to cut out extraneous things and concentrate on what matters most. Surprisingly it is not essential to have a well-functioning body for the mind to survive. In fact, some people begin to come to terms with their lives only after they begin letting go of the ego's attachment to their bodies. At some point, our identification becomes less with our bodies and more with the sustaining force that strengthens us.

If we visit a cemetery or attend a funeral, the message is always the same. Our final being is not limited to our present bodies.

How do we receive this message? The answer involves love and sacrifice. We all have the capacity to experience joy — actively pursuing love and sacrifice is what releases that true joy.

## The Bliss Of Quiet Heroism
* * * * * * *

I once knew a middle-aged man who had crawled out on a frozen lake to rescue a young person who had fallen through the ice. This man was only a passerby who did not know the young man. He was not able to say exactly why he had responded as he did. There were no long tree limbs, no ladders nor anything available to use in such a rescue. He walked right out to the edge of the ice, risking his own life in the process. There were no other people in the vicinity to help. It was also possible that the young man was actually attempting suicide and wanted to make death appear to be an accident. The young man was not crying out for help.

The passerby could have looked the other way and rationalized that perhaps the boy was already dead. In spite of these reservations, alone and unaided, the man crawled directly out to the edge of the ice, took off his coat, put it around the boy's neck, and pulled him to safety. He then administered CPR and eventually the boy started breathing. By this time, the authorities had arrived and were able to assist.

The hero did not feel like a hero at all. In fact, he did not even feel that he had done anything unusually brave. In talking with him about this event, I discovered that he actually felt he had absolutely no choice in risking his own life to save that of the young boy. I have often reflected upon *why* this man was willing to risk his own life, as well as the financial and perhaps emotional security of his own children and family, for a stranger he had never seen before and who did not seek his help. What led him to believe that he had no choice in the matter? What kind of internal reasoning prompted him to act so selflessly?

Schopenhauer believed we live partly in our own realm and partly within a context affecting or being affected by everyone else. He believed that a constant action and interaction exists between the forces of our physical and mental presences and the forces of the physical and mental presence of everything and everyone else around us. He probably would have found the middle-aged man's rescue story an example of one's individual self interacting or acting upon the collective community of all of our mental selves. This view of collective consciousness has been called cosmic consciousness by some writers. The peak of cosmic consciousness occurs when, for a moment, we experience a sense of ultimately belonging with the forces of all else in this world.

The rescuer said that during the episode he felt more "alive" than at any other time he could recall. He confessed that he "relished" that experience, not because he was being a "hero," but because he was doing something which made him feel alive and functional.

Many other people who have been involved in similar life-threatening experiences speak of terror or rage, but also admit they felt totally alive for the first time, a feeling which surpassed any awareness of fear.

My combat experiences in Vietnam and the experiences of many veterans I have counseled confirm the power of those peak moments. Although many of us went through terrible circumstances, we would still like to regain, capture and hold those feelings of being truly alive. Nothing seems to compare.

## The Knowingness Of The Mature Personality
\* \* \* \* \* \* \*

What exactly is it that exemplifies a truly mature and healthy personality? Is there an ideal personality type that we could strive toward? There are many highly individualistic parts to our personalities, but I find certain characteristics consistent with maturity. Having these characteristics suggests manifestation of the positive power of the sixth chakra. In maturity the power of the mind is used in a flexible, intuitive way. Many sides of a question can be seen. Men and women become wise and caring as they grow in knowledge. They are conscious of their influence and the effect they have on others and use their power with awareness and with good intent.

## Directions Of Conscious Maturity
* * * * * * *

Certain predictable shifts of direction indicate that we are becoming mature. They are good goals to strive toward.

### From Ego Enhancement To Service

Truly mature people are not overly concerned about the physical. They appear to others as individually authentic, not phony, unreal, contrived or superficial. There is a definite shift of emphasis away from enhanced social self and toward a stronger spiritual self. An authentically mature person enjoys fine things, looking nice and having a circle of friends, yet their central interest has shifted from ego enhancement toward service to others and general spiritual concerns.

### From Material Ambition To Spirituality

The primary goal of mature persons is to be ambitious for "goodness' sake" rather than just for money, fame or position. A mature person does not go to extremes. An extreme would be having such high ideals spiritually or materially that they can never be reached.

### From Individualism To Community

The mature person has a sense of community with those they perceive as striving to be good. Chief Joseph of the Nez Perce Indian tribe said that all good people are members of the same tribe. The feeling of relatedness to other members of the tribe who are attempting, in their own ways, to improve our world releases positive power into the universe.

## From Reaction To Proaction

Mature persons are not easy to goad into inappropriate reactions. They are self-possessed and control their emotions, not rigidly but with ease. Their priorities are in order, yet the truly mature person can be flexible when it comes to understanding others' priorities.

## From Self-Centeredness To Empathy

The ability to be empathic and understanding of others improves as we grow, and we become more kind, faithful and loyal to others. The real reason we have empathy for others is not to understand them, but to be able to pray for them. Empathy is not sympathy. It is being able to sustain intimacy, to listen with a third ear, to see with a third eye. When the empathic response is strong, we can determine another's feelings and identify so strongly with the other's experience *we actually share it*.

## From Worrying To Humor

Humor runs deep in healthy personalities and allows us to see life for what it is. The mature person attempts to understand the mystery and the tragedy of life, but also recognizes its hilarity, absurdity and incomprehensibility at the same time. Circus clowns remind us that life is simultaneously tragic and humorous. In moments when life is difficult, seeing the humor of existence is a vital component of healthy survival.

I have always enjoyed a good joke and frequently ask my friends and patients to tell me their favorite. A person's best joke usually reveals his underlying belief about life.

## From Chaos To Perfection

Every sage and philosopher has discussed living in a state of perfection. Few in the Western world attain this stage, which represents the full blossoming of all our chakra energies or subtle powers of mind. In perfection, forgiveness and love are more important than achievement, material possessions or even your own feelings. It is a state of being, not an action, though it may invoke plenty of action. Perfection is unconditional love, best summed up in the phrase "love your enemies." To return evil for evil is evil. To return good for good is human. To return good for evil is Divine. Living in a state of unconditional love is the epitome of human development.

# Meditation For Wisdom And Understanding

This meditation reinforces our ability to think and to make good decisions. It helps us to become wise, to understand various aspects of any problem or situation. Repeated practice helps to strengthen our thinking ability and allows us to easily direct our will to a higher level of functioning and purpose.

*Claim:* I will use my creative thinking ability to gain success in every worthwhile project that I undertake. There is no task too difficult for me to master.

*Affirm:* I will sow seeds of wisdom, health, prosperity and happiness. Today I will plow the garden of life with my new efforts at understanding. I will water the seeds with self-confidence and faith and will wait for the Divine to give me the rightful harvest.

*Read:* "Everyone that asketh receiveth; and he that seeketh findeth" (Matthew 7:8).

**Meditation:** Close your eyes, take a few deep breaths and imagine a very brilliant indigo-colored light emanating from the space between your eyebrows. See this light reaching down to the lower chakras, blending with them and pushing very gently up and out the top of your head. See this light spiraling about your head in an easy way that allows you to relax and to clear your mind.

When your breathing becomes deep and regular, let your eyes roll up into your head and repeat, "I am God's child, therefore I am knower of all things." Repeat this for three minutes to the rhythm of your breath, four counts inhaled and eight counts exhaled. Pay attention to the relaxing and cleansing action of this light energy throughout your head.

# 9 Connect With The Divine

## *The Seventh Step To Personal Power*

T he seventh step to personal power is one we
cannot take alone. In the first six steps, we
develop inherent qualities of mind common to
all normal human beings. Our personal power
to create opportunities and to make intelligent
choices comes from learning to access, nurture
and use our gifts. The important lessons of
life's journey are about becoming our best
selves and making intelligent choices to achieve
a high level of personal development. I believe
the saying, "be the best of whatever you are,"
holds profound truth. We are all capable of
personal excellence in some way.

The seventh and highest step represents communion between our best selves and the Divine source of all existence. The seventh chakra is located at the crown of the head and is called *Sahasrara*, which means *thousand-petaled* in Sanskrit. It is usually pictured as a thousand-petaled lotus which may be white to symbolize the light of universal consciousness or purple to indicate the highest, most "royal" level of human consciousness. The lotus symbolizes the infinite sensitivity and strength of a flower, open to sunlight, starshine and the dew of morning. It shows us that, in the same way, we can fully open ourselves to Divine intervention. One Hindu teacher says the seventh chakra is the crown of human existence, the opening into which God can pour grace.

The number seven has had mystical significance throughout time, appearing in rites of magic, miracles and purification. It appears in the Bible more than 650 times in every book from Genesis to Revelation. Noah waited seven days after the flood to land, for example. Jesus fed the crowd with seven loaves. In the ancient world numbers were sacred clues to the nature of the universe, and seven was generally the prime sacred number found in magic incantations in Egypt and Mesopotamia. Whenever ancient people heard the word seven they sensed the power of the Divine.

Who can describe the Divine? When we study the chakra system, we find that much more is written about the first six chakras than about the Sahasrara. One teacher of meditation suggests that if we really want to get something done in this world we should meditate on the heart; if we meditate on the crown chakra, there is a danger that we might lose our stability in life. I doubt that Westerners trying to create opportunities to better their lives will spend so much time meditating that they lose touch with reality. That's certainly not my intention when I use the chakra system as a model for personal development.

When you establish a connection with a Divine source, it's not important what you call the source. Whether or not you have anything to do with established churches or organized religion, you can tap into the great creative resource housed within your spiritual self. In this book I speak of God and prefer to describe Him as the Holy Spirit, which reflects my belief system. I believe that His Holy Spirit works in our lives and that we can tap into His power as a source of inexhaustible energy and creativity. This is only possible if we allow ourselves to be as open and receptive as the thousand-petaled lotus.

## Relationship With The Divine Source
* * * * * * *

All relationships are temporary except our relationship with God. It is the only everlasting relationship we will ever have, even though our concept of God may change during our lifetime. There has been much debate about what constitutes a healthy relationship with the Holy Spirit. Some people state that their relationship with God is entirely unlike other relationships, even very close ones.

Many people pray, conduct pilgrimages, read books, take courses, study the Bible and other holy books and attend worship services of all kinds in an effort to experience the Divine. For the very devout, an ongoing relationship with a Divine source is the essence of life, the most cherished aspect of their being. The relationship you maintain with God plays a large part in enhancing every aspect of your development.

## Concepts Of God
* * * * * * *

For 35 years I have taught Sunday school classes to adults and children of all ages. I present the image of God to children in ways they can understand and relate to their experience. Whether it is an image of a kindly older man in the sky, an angel or a loving shepherd who faithfully watches over His little lambs, my presentation of God depends upon the age of the children and their ability to understand relationships. If you think back to how your own concept of God has changed over the years, you'll notice how it has evolved from early childhood ideas. I often encounter adults who haven't updated their notions of God and are still at the level of sixth-grade theology.

Our beliefs in God tend to reflect our beliefs about ourselves and the nature of reality. There is God the critical and loving parent, God the rescuer, God the martyr, God the warrior and the Earth Mother Goddess. People tend to change their ideas to make their relationship with God meet their needs at a given time. Unless they understand at least the possibility of intimacy, it is difficult to conceptualize a loving, caring God who interacts with them personally. To some extent, we tend to believe about God what we experience in our relationships with others.

Relationships with our family of origin are the raw material for our experiences with God. As we grow up and mature emotionally, we begin to differentiate our feelings and view our human relationships in a more sophisticated way. At the same time our relationship with God may remain static, though there is the potential for it to become more dynamic and spiritually mature.

In a cultural context, beliefs about God may reflect the ascendancy of women and of traditionally feminine qualities. Some churches now pray to Father-Mother God, others may be dedicated to a goddess. In India gods and goddesses are worshipped equally as different manifestations of the Self. Lakshmi is the beautiful goddess of wealth and wisdom.

Perhaps there is an inborn spiritual part of us that needs a relationship with God. Some of us feel a mysterious *calling* to it at some time in our lives. If we have not experienced an intensely intimate relationship with an-

other person, family or community, we may never feel the
need for a personal relationship with God.

## How Do We Experience God?
* * * * * * *

My grandparents had a well-loved parrot named Polly
who was just like a member of the family. I recall vividly
how my father lifted me up to watch her in her cage. Polly
was such a significant member of our family that a written
history of the bird was kept, along with some of her
feathers, in the family Bible. When I learned to read I was
astonished to find out she had died six months before I
was born! I had been told about Polly and had seen the
cage in the basement. From this evidence I had created
live-parrot memories.

I was so fascinated with having created a memory for
myself that I tried it out on my mother. I hoped to get her
to remember something that had not actually happened. I
spoke with her very earnestly about an incident I had con-
cocted out of thin air, enthusiastically relating the tale to
her and prodding her for not remembering something so
obviously important to me. I made up a meeting with a
man at the grocery store who was an old friend of my
father's. I said he had told us stories about things he and
Dad had done together when they were boys. This conver-
sation had supposedly taken place in front of Mom. I talked
about it repeatedly and kept asking my mother who the
man was. Finally she came up with a name. She had begun
to relive an experience that never actually happened.

And so I learned very early in life that we can have
vivid, erroneous memories. Our minds can also alter information remarkably over a period of time. The more we
talk about experiences, either real or imagined, the more
real they become in our minds. Eventually we develop
memory traces which facts do not support. Children are
good at inventing imaginary friends, a fantasy process
that may lead to artistic creation.

In the same way, we can create our own image of God from experiences we think are religious — though they may not stem from a Divine source at all. We invent the God we want or need or think we should have, but our version may be quite different from the unfathomable mystery that God is. It's useful to ask yourself whether you are experiencing the God you created through your own thoughts and feelings or you are actually experiencing God in a direct way.

When Paul, a devout Jew, experienced God on the road to Damascus, he could never return to his old life. In the same way, when ordinary people suddenly experience God or become enlightened with a revelation, their lives are dramatically changed. Even today many people have profound religious experiences. They report they were not trying to have such an experience, but they were primed for it. Perhaps they were struggling with a decision or searching for wholeness and were not content to let their broken lives deteriorate further. They were feeling desperate enough to be open to the possibility of Divine intervention. Desperation is often the forerunner of an encounter with the Divine.

In early Jewish temples, God was said to be in the inner sanctum sanctorum — the Holiest of the Holies. Imagine the Romans' surprise when they ran in and found a completely empty room. The true essence of God cannot be represented by anything fancy or showy. Rather it is communicated by the still, small voice within. God's work in our lives brings us the ability to notice and appreciate the subtle inner voices and visions and opportunities that arise there. The gift of discernment helps us know whether they are from our Higher Power. For this we need to develop a spiritual practice of prayer and meditation. Prayer is talking to God, meditation is listening.

Besides developing a spiritual practice, is there anything we can do to predispose ourselves to experiencing the Divine? We hear reports of out-of-body experiences, deep trances, physical and psychological healings, and these are equated with Divine intervention. I am not convinced that such phenomena have anything to do with the Divine at all. Much of it may be the power of suggestion.

If you wish to determine whether your dream, hunch, vision, song or other message is inspired by God, you can use the following indicators.

## Is This From God Or Me?
\* \* \* \* \* \* \*

I've had the opportunity to speak with holy people of different faiths all over the world, and I've made it a point to ask them how we can know whether insights come from God. Their answers have a certain consistency, suggesting five ways to tell the difference between information coming from within and messages coming from a spiritual source outside ourselves.

The first sign that communication is from a spirit source is that it may come in an "if-then" mode. God, or the Holy Spirit, generally delineates choices rather than directly telling people what to do. In this way, God seems to give options and consequences. The idea is that if you do A, then B will happen. If you do C, then D will happen. This is very different from taking advice from a friend or from your own ego. For example, the hero of *Field of Dreams* was told, "If you build it, they will come." He finally built it, and they came. If he had then become involved at the level of ego and decided that anything he built would attract good spirits and people, he could have gone very wrong on his next project. Listening to Divine inspiration requires a humble mind, free of ego.

Secondly, holy people often experience a sense of humor in the spirit source. This humor is very individualistic in nature. In other words, the funny things that are said will only be understood and amusing to the receiver. This spiritual comedian only does his routine for you, leaving

those around you out of the joke. Voltaire once said that
God was a comedian playing to an audience that is afraid
to laugh! One friend reports a voice inside her head inton-
ing, "Trust yourself," and then as an aside, "And while
you're at it, trust your cat, too." She promptly went home
and let out her house cat with no unfortunate results.

A third indication of a spiritual source is that it will
often seem to be communicating to you in a different
part of your body, head or brain than other communication you usually receive. The communication enters just
over your right or left eyebrow, or some location not
normally experienced.

A fourth characteristic of spiritual communication is an
element of surprise. The revelation will not appear as you
might have thought. You would not expect it to be just
the way it is. Often the communication will come as a
sudden insight, epiphany, or an "aha!" experience straight
out of nowhere.

Fifth, a spiritual communication often contains a play
on words, or something in symbolic form that is hard to
discern. When I teach groups to pray, I ask them to go out
by themselves and select an object, something which
seems to be special or strikingly beautiful. I then encourage them to start to think and brainstorm about the qualities of that object and permit that object to speak to
them. I then ask them to bring back the object, if possible,
and share it with the group.

Once I was meditating in a forest near a small stream.
A walnut that had fallen into the river caught my attention
and I was transfixed, watching it go around and around in
an eddy near the bank. Suddenly I realized that I was
caught up in a pattern of behavior that had me going
around in circles too. I hadn't recognized it until the symbolic lesson of the walnut in the stream came into my
conscious awareness.

When we allow ourselves free-form meditation, when
we are alone and the world is quiet, God may speak to

us. We need only listen. In the Bible and in other holy literature, God talks to people in their dreams. It is a possibility for all of us. That is why it is very important to analyze our dreams. They are a rich source of guidance, offering options and explanations, revealing meaning and knowledge.

Finally, we can experience the Divine by learning to think theologically.

## Theological Reflection
*  *  *  *  *  *  *

When we "reflect," we look back and examine an experience. Reflection may be deliberate or involuntary. Theological reflection involves deliberately examining an experience to discover a direction for living a more "holy" or spiritually based life.

Serious reflection is exacting work involving understanding, emotion and telling ourselves the truth. In theological reflection we involve our spiritual nature as we open our hearts and minds to the possibilities of God's call to us. Through this process we are better able to find a positive way to live with the ambiguity and brokenness of our world.

There are four primary sources of knowledge used during theological reflection. The *action* source takes into account all that we experience in life. Past and present experiences and feelings are based in this source. When we find ourselves making statements such as "I feel . . .," "I remember . . .," or "I grew up . . .," we are speaking from the Action source.

The *position* source encompasses our opinions, beliefs and attitudes. These positions can appear in the most casual of conversations as well as in tough contract negotiations. "I believe . . .," "All men are . . .," "In my opinion . . ." are all examples of a person speaking from the Position source.

The *culture* source incorporates everything from tradition, political affiliation, movies, books, museums, educational systems, professional ethics, sexual and behavioral mores to common sense. Phrases like "My mother always told me . . .," "It's a fact that . . .," or "Nice people generally . . ." have the culture source as a base.

Finally, there is the *tradition* source. It could be considered the public content of faith: scriptures, church history, creeds, dogma, doctrines, rituals, architecture and twentieth-century theology. We are speaking from this source when we say "Jesus said . . .," "The Torah tells us . . .," or "Zen teaches us . . ."

When we combine these four sources, it is easy to understand why no two people share exactly the same viewpoint. Our experience and learning are ours exclusively, despite the common threads that bind our lives together.

### *10 Methods For Theological Reflection*

1. Remember a moment when your beliefs or assumptions were challenged. Write it down.
2. List the shifts of action in the story. Focus on one.
3. Recall thoughts and feelings you experienced at that time.
4. Write down this information.
5. Think of a metaphor that parallels this story. (For example, your life after divorce might conjure up images of a roller coaster suddenly out of control.)
6. From the viewpoint of each of the four sources, action, position, culture and tradition, describe your metaphor:
   A. Can you describe the world?
   B. What is negative?
   C. Where is judgment?
   D. Where is God?
   E. What would be a cause for celebration?
7. Think back to Tradition. What story or parable might correspond to your metaphor?

8. Examine the four source positions, and then state your own position (on paper).
9. Identify insights you have gained or new questions this examination may have initiated.
10. Decide how this may relate to your approach to similar situations in the future.

This process takes a lot of work and thought, but it is well worth it. To elaborate a bit, the first step involves taking any event, problem or situation that is of concern to you and thinking of it as a metaphor. In other words, what do you feel like, or what can the situation, event or problem be compared to in terms of a story, an object or any kind of "happening"? Keep thinking until you come up with the metaphor that depicts how "life is" for you in this situation.

Let me give you an example and work through some of the situations for you. Recently a woman I know had a great learning experience. Her husband had died of cancer. Her message was that the time had come to clean out his closet, as well as her own. She kept thinking about what would be an appropriate meaning for her situation. She came up with the idea that it would be the metaphor of leaving home for the first time.

First she wrote the message down in a section entitled "life is." She then started reflecting on some of the things that were negative about it. Some of the things she listed were: losing the memory of her husband, giving away or throwing out too many clothes of her own and other negative aspects of her activity. The third aspect of the metaphor was "what could go wrong in this situation" for her. She came up with items such as not having enough clothes in the future, not having something when she wanted it, such as a special garment for a special occasion. About this time, she came to the realization that what she was really afraid of was being needy.

She did not actually need anything except the companionship of her husband whom she missed a great deal. Her greatest fear, then, was that she would be needy and not able to get what she required in the future. This woman discovered that what she really was afraid of was fear. This fear was perpetuating the situation and also the bad feelings surrounding it.

The final part of this plan is to determine what sense of celebration might be applicable in this situation. She decided that life is a cycle of gaining and losing, and that the option she would take would be to consider her life an adventure and to go forward onto her new path.

## Connecting With A Divine Source
*       *       *       *       *       *       *

The ideas contained in this chapter do not represent the ultimate in knowing God, for no one will ever thoroughly understand how the Divine works. I do, however, feel that these techniques can assist anyone in improving his or her relationship with God. I am also convinced that thinking about things theologically will open new doors of perception and increase the options and opportunities we can create for ourselves. Yours can be a joyful search. The great psychoanalyst, Heinz Kohut, says:

> The world of creative science is inhabited by playful people who understand that the reality that surrounds them is essentially unknowable. Realizing that they can never get at "the" truth, only at analogizing approximations, they are satisfied to describe what they see from various points of view, and to explain it as best they can in a variety of ways.

The depths of God are truly unknowable. We delude ourselves if we claim we have God or the Divine in our grasp. We need to adopt a spirit of joy and playfulness in our attempts to comprehend the Divine.

God and the Holy Spirit work in unique and different ways for all of us. But when we know that our internal communication is coming from a spiritual source, lasting change can take place.

# Meditation For Aligning With Divine Will

Meditate to surrender your personal will to the will of the Divine. Repeated practice of this meditation will help strengthen and align your will with spiritual direction.

*Claim:* In God's blessed light I will remain forever with Him.

*Affirm:* I turn my will and my life over to the God of my understanding. I am open to the gentle wisdom of Divine guidance.

*Read:* "The wisdom that comes down from above is essentially something pure; it is also peaceable, kindly and considerate; it is full of mercy and shows itself by doing good; nor is there any trace of partiality or hypocrisy in it" (James 3:17).

*Meditation:* This meditation is designed to help align your own purposes with that of the Divine. Close your eyes and take a few deep breaths. Imagine that your breath is moving from the soles of your feet to the top of your head. Experience a very brilliant violet-to-white light surrounding your entire head and reaching down and drawing up all of the brilliant crystal lights from your lower chakras up into your head area. See the white light beginning to rise like a fountain, which gently sprinkles healing white light completely over and through your body.

When your breathing becomes deep and regular, let your eyes roll up into your head and repeat, "I am part of the light of the world."

Repeat this for three minutes to the rhythm of your breath, four counts inhaled and eight counts exhaled. Pay close attention and enjoy the feeling of the energy moving from the lower chakras up and out the top of your head, covering your whole body in a brilliant rainbow of light and healing energy.

# 10 Taking The 7 Steps To Personal Power

## *How They Work Together*

I n the following story John and Mary are com-
posites of many clients I have worked with
over the last 20 years. While their story is not
a real case history, it closely parallels the actual
course of change for many people.

### The First Step
★ ★ ★ ★ ★ ★ ★

John and Mary were in their mid-thirties,
had an average life, but were bored, in debt,
and their children seemed to need less attention than before. They each had bouts of mild
depression and were sometimes short-tem-
pered and fatigued. They were not as intensely

involved with each other as they once were, and each considered having an affair. Maybe they should divorce. Move to another town. They couldn't really put their fingers on a specific problem, but had what I call the "Get-a-new-life" syndrome.

When they came to my office they took their first step to personal power — they claimed the power within. In fact, when they called for their first appointment, they *claimed*:

1. Their right to get help
2. Their hope and belief that something might change
3. Their willingness to find an answer
4. Their willingness to be empowered

## The Second Step To Personal Power
* * * * * * *

During the first appointment, I listened to them explain their situation, then asked them to imagine what kind of outcome would be acceptable. When they answered that very important question, they took a rudimentary second step to personal power — *create what you need*. When John and Mary began to use the creative power of the second step to imagine an acceptable outcome, it opened the rusty locks of their imaginations. Many more creative ideas would be set forth before they had generated enough options to make good decisions, but they were on the way. The second step had been taken.

## The Third Step
* * * * * * *

After a few sessions, some of the fears that were limiting their lives had emerged, and they were able to work with them. They began to be able to express their emotions to each other without getting carried away with emotion, thus initiating the third step to personal power,

*cultivate emotional balance.* I helped them work through negative emotions of anger, fear and negative beliefs in order
to cultivate the emotional balance the third step to personal power requires. As we took this third step, we kept
the energy of the first two steps in play as well, claiming
and affirming their will and right to an interesting successful life and their ability to create workable ideas. As
we worked through their negative emotions, more emotional energy became available on the positive side. Sparks
of enthusiasm became evident.

But there were still buried angers and resentments to
work through. They had submerged small and large hurts
they had caused each other. In the depths of their unconscious minds, these hurts were linked to earlier pains
from their families of origin. We had to do some deep and
painful work to bring them into the light and discharge
the negative emotions they had accumulated.

## The Fourth Step
\* \* \* \* \* \* \*

The work of opening the heart might have been difficult, painful or threatening had we started with deep
analysis on our first appointments, but because we laid
the groundwork of developing the foundational strengths
of the first three chakras and the personal energies they
represent, John and Mary had the resources to get over
the hurdles of deep pain. They were able to rekindle the
heartfelt love they had for each other and find the willingness to forgive. In the process of freeing their hearts,
they began to find enough available energy to *set their
hearts on change.* They began to enjoy the work we were
doing together and began to come up with some interesting options to overcome their boredom. Their unconscious minds were getting messages of hope, optimism
and belief in the possibility of positive outcomes, and

began responding with powerful positive ideas, feelings, moods and energy levels.

By this time both Mary and John felt much more energetic, and Mary, who had been overweight, lost her interest in overeating even though dieting was never discussed in our sessions. As forgiveness entered their lives, they could let go, not only of hidden memories of the past, but of bad habits of the present. They were excited that their children seemed to want to spend more time with them. Laughter and physical intimacy were returning to their lives on a fairly regular basis.

# The Fifth Step
*★ ★ ★ ★ ★ ★ ★*

When John and Mary began to release their fears and antagonisms, they began to *go with their inner voices.* As they developed the ability to listen to the voice of their hearts, they also became better, more attentive listeners for each other. This led to being able to speak with each other with much more intimacy than either had dreamed possible before. As their level of communication became more solid, they spoke more easily to each other of their hopes and dreams. Their dreams began to look and sound very real. John had always wanted to play the violin, but never felt it was appropriate. After all, he was the responsible, macho breadwinner for his family. The violin would be a waste of time. Mary encouraged his musical interests and came up with some of her own. She had been interested in local politics and decided to volunteer at party headquarters. Soon she found a real niche for herself doing fundraising. She confided to John that she would like to run for the school board some day.

You see how this couple's life took unexpected turns. They had come into therapy thinking in terms of divorce, moving to another city, quitting their jobs. Within a few months they had found new depth in their relationship and new connections with their family and their community. Their therapy had taken unexpected turns. Without tossing out the old, they were creating wonderful opportunities to enrich and enjoy their lives.

## The Sixth Step
* * * * * * *

Confidence grew. John and Mary became more self-assured as they experienced small wins. They enjoyed themselves and felt that life would sustain them. Still, they had the sense that they could have more if they wanted it. They began to *know the power within.* They began to understand that to reach any major change in their lives they would have to have very clear intentions. They began to focus on long-term goals and formulate realistic plans for reaching them. Previously they had built castles in the air, now they were building firm foundations under them. They delineated a plan of action complete with timetable and thought through how action steps would be accomplished. They participated as partners, each bringing their greatest strengths to the project. They had many good ideas, options and choices.

## The Seventh Step
* * * * * * *

When John and Mary learned to trust the possibility of Divine guidance and let God's grace into their lives, they relaxed noticeably. Taking time for prayer and meditation on a regular basis was a difficult practice to start, but when they became established in their spiritual practice they felt truly *connected with the Divine,* and blessings began to flow. They brought to their lives their best thinking, most heartfelt feelings, joy, enthusiasm and emotional honesty.

Do they still have problems? Of course. Do they still come for counseling? Hardly ever. The seven-step system is a natural way to align your life with God's plan for you, with your highest and best self. You can use it on your own, as John and Mary did, to bring relief and improvement to any situation.

## Hitting Paydirt
★ ★ ★ ★ ★ ★ ★

When you develop your personal power and harmonize it with the universal energy of God, you can reach your highest good. Reaching that level of excellence is an ongoing process that keeps us vital and interested in life. Our notions of what constitutes success may change, our interests shift, our levels of compassion and caring increase as we go through this process.

Being fully alive in the moment will probably supplant any need you have to conform and live up to others' expectations.

In my part of Oklahoma almost everyone gets into the oil business sooner or later, at least as an investor. One large oil company is referred to as the Total Death Corporation. Its employees file into their offices at exactly 8:30 in the morning and file out again at 5:00. They have opted for security and a pension, and in exchange traded in their aliveness and ability to choose. They really think they are getting something in return for marching in lock-step to the company's tune, but I don't agree. So-called security is a seductive myth.

The interesting people in the oil business are the wildcatters, who combine their intuition with their knowledge. They get geological surveys made, lease land and oilfield equipment, hire rowdies and roustabouts to man the drilling rigs and sometimes bring in a gusher. They take risks, have fun, make money, suffer losses — and they go on. They have an excitement about their work and life in general that the people in the offices of large corporations can't begin to imagine.

Should we become wildcatters of life? Not necessarily. But when we learn to develop all of our God-given abilities and mental powers, learn to trust ourselves and God, we can choose to be wildcatters if we want to be. We can create any opportunities that suit us. The challenges of life become a joy.

I truly believe that as we look at our lives and accept the challenge of change and renewal, we will become those people we dreamed of becoming. Our choices are as big as our dreams, and our dreams are as real as our ability to follow them.

GRACE and PEACE

# CHAPTER
# 11 Are You Out Of Options?

## *51 Things To Do When Nothing Else Works*

**1.** Ask yourself, "Why does this keep happening to me over and over again?" Your answer will lead you to understand the constructive and destructive behavioral patterns that play an important part in your life.

**2.** Ask yourself, "What am I angry or hurt about?" When someone is depressed or in a bad mood, it's probably because they're angry about an issue they haven't addressed. Imagine the hurt as the core of an onion, hidden by layers of false defenses and negative feelings. It can only be discovered when we release our negative thoughts and do some internal exploration. When we forgive, it frees us from the responsibility of carrying this anger around any longer.

177

**3.** Ask yourself, "How would my life be different without this problem?" This is a way of discovering what your problem does for you. In your own imagination ask your symptom what is going on, the same way you might ask a child with a stomachache what his stomach needs.

**4.** Consult with a colleague or friend. No matter how well we know ourselves, we have our blind spots. Talking about our ideas with someone else helps clarify what is actually happening.

**5.** Ask yourself 20 questions. What's your favorite color, fairy tale, movie, song, book, place? What's your favorite car, three wishes, joke or saying? Use your answers to make a hypothesis about the nature of the person who gave these answers.

**6.** Talk about your feelings of failure and learn to recognize how they can teach you a lesson. Failure is never failure if it leads to learning. It is only failure if we do not learn.

**7.** Ask your internal family for advice. Communicate with all your different parts to find a way to improve your situation.

**8.** Get your family members into the problem-solving process. Your family are supposed to be your best friends and support group. Enlist their help.

**9.** Try polarities. Do the opposite of what is expected of you. Some polar opposites are, for example, blaming versus placating or being super-reasonable instead of irrational. Whenever you respond in the same old way, it means you have become too narrow in your judgments.

**10.** Sleep, withdraw temporarily or go on a trip to get away. Simply get away from a problem until you have the strength to handle it.

**11.** Use the collapsing technique. This is a technique that helps you put opposite situations or opinions together, then generate compromise. Imagine holding one issue in the right hand, another in the left. Then put the two palms together. This will let you "get into" and experience each side of an argument.

**12.** Think about how you could make things worse. Determine that you really do have power in a situation. At least you can influence it, if only in a negative way. This maneuver may be exactly what is needed to break up patterns of negative thinking and open the door to positive ideas.

**13.** Write down your experiences. Keep a journal only when you feel it's appropriate instead of keeping a daily diary. Looking back over your feelings helps you understand why you were emotional in the past and how you feel or think now.

**14.** Be brave. Go back to square one. Sometimes when we are working on an issue, we temporarily get confused or lost. Reflecting on the beginning helps us remember what we're trying to do, then take a fresh look at what is actually happening.

**15.** Try medication. Sometimes using approved medication can give you the temporary strength you need to get your feelings or anxiety under control. Discuss this option with your physician.

**16.** Do the "biblical" thing. Often when people are in an ethical dilemma, an answer is already waiting in their theological value system.

**17.** Mentally change your history. Imagine something good happened to you, even if something bad actually happened. Superimpose the good scene over the bad one you actually experienced until the entire image becomes a positive one.

**18.** Learn to relax and meditate. This is extremely important. There are a lot of books that can teach you how to meditate. Choose whichever one works best for you.

**19.** Accept the really honest truth. The most important thing in problem-solving is to know the truth. No matter what the truth is, people can handle it better than they can handle a lie. Ask yourself whether you are truly being honest in your self-examination.

**20.** Use acupressure to relieve symptoms. Acupressure, shiatsu, reflexology and other psychophysical techniques can be used to relieve pressure and pain. Go to a practitioner or learn to do them on yourself. Many fairly accurate and comprehensive books are available. These therapies are the treatments of choice in the Far East.

**21.** Create a guided fantasy or project your problem onto an object. Visualize yourself walking through the woods and coming upon an unexpected situation. Decide what you can do in that situation. This will lead you to understand your motivations. Or, try projecting yourself onto an inanimate object. If your problem is your relationship with an in-law, put the in-law in a chair (in your imagination) and talk to that person. Then move into the in-law's chair and talk back to yourself as if you were now that person. You will generate some new options, learn to empathize and have better encounters with that person in a real situation.

**22.** Pray. Praying for others, especially those who have hurt you and who you feel are your enemies, is very powerful. In a prayer from the heart, ask for the ability to cope with the situation.

**23.** Learn what you can from an object. Go outdoors or sit in your own room and look at something interesting. Study it and then simply describe the object. Anything you say about it beyond its physical description represents your projections.

**24.** Make a contract with your symptoms. Use the technique described in Chapter 7 to discover what your symptoms are doing for you.

**25.** Contemplate on a verse or saying. As you begin to ponder on it, you will discover its implication and find a deeper meaning than you did before. Use this technique to guide you in understanding your problems and help you generate some choices for yourself.

**26.** Assume you deliberately created this problem. You are making this assumption to determine whether your situation is a form of self-protection. You may simply be creating a defense mechanism to save you from an imagined fear.

**27.** Go to therapy. Do it for your own growth. A good therapist will help you learn a lot about yourself. The information you gain is well worth the time and money invested.

**28.** Discuss increasing your sessions or terminating therapy. Sometimes this will motivate you to get moving on a program of success. Certainly if you feel you are making insufficient progress in handling your situation or in creating new opportunities, you need to discuss this with your therapist.

**29.** Stop all substance abuse. The word "substance" here includes alcohol, nicotine, caffeine, sugar, legal and illegal drugs. Avoiding these substances can make a real difference in how you feel, think and process information.

**30.** Get a pet. Having a pet can contribute to your well-being, longevity and happiness.

**31.** Spend more time with your children individually. The time spent individually with a child often helps bring out our inner child. Any time spent individually, especially with our own children, will give us clues as to how we actually do things since children are a reflection of us and our ways of behaving.

**32.** Go to church or somewhere to worship. The spiritual strength you get through worship is invaluable. It is very important to get comfortable with the idea of meeting your spiritual needs.

**33.** Forgive. This spiritual work is one of the most important exercises anyone can do. Lack of forgiveness can immobilize you. When we forgive others, we can move ahead in our own growth. Revenge is deadly for both the attacker and the avenger.

**34.** Stay up late at night once a week. Variation in routine alleviates depression and provides time to enjoy solitude.

The time can be spent constructively in such pursuits as writing a journal or doing something else you enjoy.

**35.** Eat a healthy diet. We know we should, yet few of us actually do eat healthy foods. When we eat the right foods, our internal and external lives work better.

**36.** Visit an old friend. Spending time with supportive, loving people who care for you usually helps. It's a relief from the present situation and your friends can help you create new options you may have missed.

**37.** Write your own funeral service. This is one way people with a heightened fear of death or loss can face the fear. Confronting the idea that they ultimately will die seems to lessen the hold death has over their lives. Being with people at the time of their death has taught me that people do not die in pain or fear. This is a perception created in movies and novels that does not hold true in real life.

**38.** Learn self-hypnosis. There are several good textbooks on self-hypnosis and Silva mind control that can teach us to relax, learn to be more comfortable with ourselves or simply get some symptom relief.

**39.** Go back to when your problems began. Think back to when you first felt some kind of bad feeling and return to that situation in your mind. This may take a while, but when you go back, you may be able to update the decisions you made.

**40.** Cry. Crying is therapeutic. Men usually receive a great deal of relief when they cry despite society's strong injunctions against this display of emotions.

**41.** Scream. It sometimes helps. An especially good place to do it is in your car with the windows rolled up and the radio blaring.

**42.** Take full responsibility for whatever happens to you. To gain control of your situation, imagine you deliberately set it up. Now ask yourself what it is that you want.

**43.** Create. This is absolutely one of the most helpful things anyone can do. Everyone has the ability to create, whether it is to draw, dance, paint, write, make something or just to abstractly play with concepts in color and design. One thing is certain: There is no other work of art just like yours. This creating is an affirmation that we are indeed unique and no duplication of us or our work can ever exist. Creating also helps us release tension and generate new options.

**44.** Write a letter. This may help you vent some of your anger if you are disappointed with someone or have something to say. If you are hesitant about sending it, write the letter anyway and later tear it up. It will make you feel better, organize your thoughts and help you communicate with that other person.

**45.** Go to your "healing place." Our "healing place" may be in our imagination, or somewhere we have spent a lot of time, either having a good time or getting support. Sometimes just being in this "healing place" will help us establish the mindset we need in order to deal with our problems and gain strength. Scarlett O'Hara's immediate decision when faced with misfortune was to return to Tara, her family home. Tara was her "healing place."

**46.** Mess up the internal video tapes. All of us have our own mental video tape library where we can pull video tapes off the shelf and immediately start rerunning them through our heads. You can get yourself into a terrible mood in a little over four seconds if you really want to. But why should you? Instead, block your tape's negative impact. Freeze it as it is going along, change the color to black and white. Make it very shiny and dub in voices of opera stars, country singers or howling dogs. You can also run it backwards, make people speak in a foreign language. Make it as unreal and ridiculous as possible. Try hard to mess up the reality of your negative tapes.

**47.** Start living by the ten/ten rule. Remember the secret of growing rich slowly: Give away ten percent and save ten percent of all that you make.

**48.** Do something every single day to move toward your number one goal. This is one of the most important things you can do for yourself. Another goal is to make sure you have clearly written down or communicated your goal to yourself.

**49.** Analyze your dreams, then ask your unconscious mind to give you an answer in your dreams. Remember to have paper and a pencil by your bed when you wake up to write down your dream.

**50.** Make up something else. You can make up something else to do using several different techniques. The first is the "soaking laundry" technique. If you will give your unconscious mind a chance to work on something, without really pushing yourself, you will eventually have a creative and good solution to any problem.

Another technique you can use is to mentally make your problem as ridiculous as you can. Carry it to the extreme and imagine both good and bad outcomes. Perhaps the most important thing to understand is that there are some middle-of-the-road circumstances you have to really work at and clarify before you can move on.

Another way to think of something else is to pick an object or a saying and see how it relates to the problem you're working on.

**51.** Use the Paired Associates/Anchoring Technique. I use this technique a lot for myself and others but it is somewhat involved. It was inspired by the ideas of the Russian researcher Ivan Pavlov.

Pavlov rang a bell while simultaneously giving dogs something to eat. He discovered the dogs started salivating when he rang the bell. This classic psychological experiment was interpreted as meaning that the sound of the bell was somehow "paired" with the dogs' expectations of food. Pavlov's experiment was one of the foundation experiments in psychology and we take his findings more or less for granted today. We know that whenever two things are associated in real life, they automatically become associated in our minds, such as salt and _____ .
Most of the time people will think of pepper. There are

thousands of these kinds of associations. The most important implication of the paired associate/anchoring technique is that we can also make associations in our other senses, too, physically as well as visually, by our sense of hearing as well as our sense of smell. For example, certain smells remind us of special places, people or things, as do certain sights and sounds.

Some of my colleagues and I have learned that this very simple principle can be used as a way of healing and gaining strength in difficult times, but it must be executed exactly the way I am describing it.

First, find a very positive strong anchor. Let's say you find it difficult to talk to your boss because you feel intimidated by him or her. In the boss's presence you feel like mush. At times like these, sit down and put yourself in a "strengthening mode" by recalling a time when you felt very much in control and accepted by other people. As you do that, take your right hand and press it in the middle of your chest gently. Do this repeatedly, perhaps three or four times, and as you do, you will literally relive that one great positive experience. You will notice that as you press on your chest, the positive experience will automatically begin to become associated with the gesture of touching your chest.

Once you have that response very well "anchored," the spot on your chest becomes a strong trigger. You can touch a "feel-good button" anytime you feel distressed, lonely, powerless or depressed. In the presence of your boss, or whenever you feel rather down, press on your chest in exactly the same spot. You will again experience the good feeling you had when you were accepted and loved.

An accountant came to me who had been caught embezzling from his corporation. He had an interview the next morning and was told if he made it through the interview all right, he would probably keep his job. If he promised to pay back what he had embezzled, there would be no criminal charges filed. I taught him the technique and he learned to make a gesture as if he were straightening his tie. This one small technique got him through the interview and has helped him a great deal ever since.

The second technique I taught him has to do with what I call the "power pose."

A local attorney, Joe Wideman, and I wrote a book on courtroom trial tactics. Part of the book was about maintaining your composure on the witness stand while under a great deal of emotional stress from being cross-examined. We found people were more at ease when they sat up straight, placed both feet flat on the floor, kept their backs straight up, their heads erect and their eyes at eye level or above. We call it the "power pose" and we have used it successfully for the last 15 years in our seminars on effective courtroom witnessing.

Often a combination of the paired associates/anchoring technique and the power pose will work best for you, and will be something you can teach others when they are in need of strength. Even as you are using these techniques, other ideas may come to you which suggest to you what to do, what to say, how to think or feel. Remember that with the power pose technique, the second you lower your eyes below the midline, you risk getting into a feeling which may not be helpful for you. Try to keep your head and eyes up.

I encourage you to try one or all of these 51 things to do when nothing else works or whenever you need to cope with an especially difficult situation. They are all field-tested options which have helped hundreds of people.

# 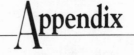ppendix

## Creative Resources

Adams, James L., **The Care And Nurturing Of Ideas,** Reading, MA: Addison Wesley, 1986.

Jones, Alex, **Creative Thought Remedies,** Marina del Rey, CA: DeVorss & Co., 1986.

Nierenberg, Gerald I., **The Art Of Creative Thinking,** New York: Simon & Schuster, 1986.

Taylor, Joshua, **Learning To Look,** Chicago: U. of Chicago Press, 1985.

## Dreams

Hall, James A., **Jungian Dream Interpretation,** Toronto: Inner City Books, 1983.

Johnson, Robert A., **Inner Work,** New York: Harper, 1986.

Williams, Strephon K., **The Jungian-Senoi Dreamwork Manual,** Berkeley, CA: Journey Press, 1986.

## Mid-life

Adler, Mortimer J., **How To Think About God,** New York: Bantam, 1980.

Frankl, Viktor E., **Man's Search For Meaning,** New York: Washington Square Press, 1962.

Singer, June, **Boundaries Of The Soul,** New York: Anchor Books, 1973.

Stein, Murray, **In Mid-life,** Dallas: Spring Pubs, 1991.

## Meditation

Brennan, Barbara Ann, **Hands Of Light,** New York: Bantam, 1988.

Goldstein, Joseph, **The Experience Of Insight,** Boston: Shambhala, 1987.

Hanh, Thich Nhat, **The Miracle Of Mindfulness,** Boston: Beacon Press, 1987.

Keyes, Ken, **Handbook To Higher Consciousness,** St. Mary, KY: Living Love Pubs., 1978.

Progoff, Ira, **The Practice Of Process Meditation,** New York: Dialogue House, 1980.

Shah, Idries, **The Way Of The Sufi,** New York: Dutton, 1970.

Short, Robert L., **A Time To Be Born — A Time To Die,** New York: Harper, 1973.

Stevens, John, **Akido,** New York: Shambhala, 1984.

# Bibliography

Berne, Eric, **Games People Play,** New York: Grove Press, 1964.

Bible Review, Washington, D.C., *Biblical Archeological Society,* June 1992, Vol. 8 No. 3, pp. 48, 49.

Bradbury, Ray, **The Martian Chronicles,** Garden City, NY: Doubleday, 1958.

Campbell, Joseph, **The Hero With A Thousand Faces,** Princeton, NJ: Princeton University Press, 1990.

Carroll, Lewis, **Alice In Wonderland,** Garden City, NY: Children's Classics.

**Diagnostic And Statistical Manual Of Mental Disorders — Revised,** Washington, D.C.: American Psychiatric Association, 1987.

Harris, Thomas, **I'm OK — You're OK, A Practical Guide To Transactional Analysis,** New York: Harper & Row, 1969.

Khan, Sufi Inayat, **The Palace of Mirrors,** Geneva: Sufi Pubs., 1935.

Kinman, Carolyn, **Education For Ministry, Common Lessons: Series "A,"** Sewanee, TN: University of the South Press, 1984.

Knapp, Stephen, **The Secret Teachings Of The Vedas,** Detroit, MI: World Relief Network, 1986.

Lansdowne, Zachary, **The Chakras And Esoteric Healing,** York Beach, ME: Samuel Weiser, Inc., 1986.

Leadbeater, C.W., **The Chakras,** London: Theosophical Pubs., 1985.

Levinson, Daniel J., **The Seasons Of A Man's Life,** New York: Alfred Knopf, 1978.

Lewis, Sinclair, **Babbitt,** NY: Buccaneer Press, reprint, 1961.

Luke, S.W., **Acupuncture Manual; A Western Approach,** New York: Marcel Dekker, Inc., 1979.

Miller, N.E. and Dollard, J., **Social Learning And Imitation,** New Haven, CT: Yale University Press, 1941.

**Nag Hammadi Library,** San Francisco, CA: Harper & Row, 1977.

**New Jerusalem Bible,** New York: Doubleday, 1985.

Pearsall, Paul, **Super Joy,** Garden City, NY: Doubleday, 1988.

Pennell, Rolla J., **The Seminar Of Acupuncture For Physicians,** Independence, MO: IPCI, Inc., 1973.

Robbins, Lois, **Waking Up In The Age Of Creativity,** Santa Fe, NM: Bear and Co., 1985.

Schopenhauer, Arthur, **The World As Will And Idea,** New York: AMS Press, 1986.

Stahl, Carolyn, **Opening To God,** Nashville, TN: Upper Room, 1977.

Sheehy, Gail, **Passages,** New York: Bantam Books, 1977.

Sivananda Radha, Swami, **Kundalini Yoga For The West,** New York: Shambhala, 1978.

Three Initiates, **The Kybalion — Hermetic Philosophy,** Chicago: Yogi Publication Society, 1912.

Toffler, Alvin, **Future Shock,** New York: Random House, 1970.

# The J. Thomas Co.

419 Fairview • Ponca City, OK 74601 • (405) 762-7251

## Tapes Available at $11.95 each

### Optimum Encounter™

This tape offers a guide to understanding how and why we allow ourselves to lead lackluster lives, and offers a step-by-step plan for breaking the mold which traps us and forces us to remain less than we could be. Side "B" of this tape is the "CPR of Mental Processing" to which any problem can be brought for resolution.

### Focused Attention

Marshal your powers of concentration. This tape allows you to focus clearly on the task at hand.

### Quick Zzzzz's™

Gain the restful, rejuvenating benefits of a complete sleep cycle in just minutes. The perfect "fix" for studying students, exhausted employees or jet-lagging travelers.

### Sleep Well

If restful sleep has eluded you, try this tape to get back on the gentle track of perfect repose.

### Meditation

Find inner peace and relaxation at their deepest levels while heightening your inner awareness. This tape provides an overview of meditation techniques relied upon by cultures over the centuries.

### Depression

Sometimes life seems to be less than we had bargained for. During these times of limitation, turn to this tape to free your spirit and regain a more positive, self-affirming perspective on your life.

### Stress

Running full-tilt through our days and nights almost seems to be the norm. This tape offers welcome relief to those on the go and those whose "go" is about gone.

### Pain Control

Hurting hampers our lives. Learning the pain control techniques on Side "B" of this tape can and will offer you a new sense of control and hope over this aspect of your life.